HOW MANY MOUNTAINS?

How Many Mountains?

Russell S. Schultze
with Willetta J. Balla

BROADMAN PRESS
Nashville, Tennessee

© Copyright 1980 · Broadman Press.
All rights reserved.
4252-72
ISBN: 0-8054-5272-9

Dewey Decimal Classification: B
Subject headings: SCHULTZE, RUSSELL S.//CEREBRAL PALSY—BIOGRAPHY
Library of Congress Catalog Card Number: 79-54921
Printed in the United States of America

DEDICATION BY RUSSELL SCHULTZE

I dedicate this book to my "super chick" Kathy, who inspired me to put my life's story together.

ACKNOWLEDGEMENT

My many thanks to my friends and relatives who, through their love, help, and encouragement, made me realize anything is possible with the Lord's help.

For obvious reasons certain names have been changed. Though several names were changed, the major events in the story are true.

Russell L. Schultz

POSSIBILITY THINKER'S CREED

When faced with a mountain
I WILL NOT QUIT! I will
keep on striving until I
climb over, find a pass
through, tunnel underneath—
or simply stay and turn the
mountain into a gold mine,
with God's help!

Dr. Robert Harold Schuller,
Founder and senior pastor,
Garden Grove Community Church,
Garden Grove, California

CONTENTS

	Introduction	13
1.	How Many Mountains?	15
2.	Movement: Wheels	17
3.	Winter: The White Tunnels	25
4.	Spring: The Winds of March—A Con Game	29
5.	Summer: Fish—Tree—Fun—Storm	33
6.	Fall: School—Outhouse—Pillsbury Panties—Redhead	39
7.	The Great Impasse: A Mountain of Plaster	49
8.	The Road Back: A Psychogenic Journey	57
9.	Time of Sadness and Discovery: School for the Handicapped	69
10.	Hopes and Dreams: My First True Love	81
11.	The Adjustment: A Search for Happiness	99
12.	The Big Tournament: Oriental Style	111
13.	Circuit Breaker: Loss—New Light—Then Love	121
14.	Heavens to Betsy: New Life—New Responsibilities	127

Introduction

Birth and death are unchanging and are experiences beyond our control, but one's life becomes an important record of individual movement and experience. Through mountains of trials, sorrows, and errors each of us climb as we build that record of our life.

And so it is that Russell S. Schultze, born a spastic, has built a remarkable record of faith and courage throughout his life. He has faced many mountains, climbed over them, found passes through some, tunneled underneath several, and has also stayed with others, turning them into a gold mine of happiness and contentment with God's help.

And now I wish to thank Dr. Robert H. Schuller for giving me permission to use his "Possibility Thinker's Creed" for this autobiography.

I also want to thank Dr. Robert J. Graham of Moline, Illinois, for his medical advice in writing this story of Mr. Schultze's life.

WILLETTA J. BALLA

1 How Many Mountains?

Maggots were spilled from a tube into my body cast which reached from my feet to my armpits.

I screamed and shuddered as the sickening activity of the maggots began consuming the dead flesh which lay beneath my three-year prison the doctors had placed me in. I begged for more narcotics. I was ten when I entered the hospital at Lincoln, Nebraska. At thirteen I became addicted to the drugs given me during my three-year hospital confinement.

As late as 1937 maggots were used to clear body casts of dead flesh in order to promote the healing of pressure ulcers. The doctors felt my cast was necessary in order to keep my muscles stretched or to keep them in their proper position.

My condition is one of motor control, a form of spastic paralysis. I have always had complete feeling throughout my body, but some of my brain cells did not develop or were destroyed at birth. The result was a reversal of motor control. For example: when I put my arm up, I'm thinking I'm putting it down. And to say the least, I am clumsy. I cannot walk, and my legs are rigid.

As I grew older my body motions became more automatic, except when I was under severe stress or strain. I still have this problem today, and even my speech is affected at times under stress. My motor control is still forever in battle with my brain.

The three years in the hospital at Lincoln, Nebraska, were a nightmare, but after struggling for two years to throw off the drug habit I acquired while in the hospital, my life picked up again.

There is no life for an addict. He can never discover or experience an apocalypse, a revelation as to what life is all about, because he is transported into nothing through his indulgence, his mind playing games of hide and seek as he struggles through a terrorizing search which leads him nowhere. Mind distorted, he sees not reality, but only a maze of wild colors and shapes that do not exist. He is carried away from reality, his experiences ending in suffering in the hours that follow as he screams and begs for more drugs.

I feel my story should begin some years after my painful drug experience, when at age twenty-nine I had an adventure which spirited me on in my search for God, peace, and happiness.

2 Movement: Wheels

Freedom was foremost in my mind. How could I—a spastic—gain the freedom I yearned for?

At this particular time in my life I was spending the summer on a small ranch nine miles from a little Arkansas town called Mena, watching over my sister's three children while she worked.

I couldn't go very far in my wheelchair, so I built a gas-driven tricycle contraption—one wheel in front and two in the back. It had a steering bar resembling a scorpion's curled-up tail, along with a hand throttle and a hand brake. I put a two-horsepower gasoline engine on the back of my little tricycle car. It was quite a machine! It wouldn't back up, but I didn't want to go backward. I wanted to be free—free of my wheelchair—free to travel and see things, climbing steep hills, my mind and eyes searching for an answer to life.

I drove my little car all over the mountain roads when I wasn't tending to my sister's children, and how many close calls I had I can't say. But the dangers I faced one particular Sunday spirited me on, and later I discovered a gold mine of love, happiness, and contentment I never dreamed possible.

Climbing mountains to some may not seem to be so exciting, but the more I drove my car up and down the steep grades, the more my desire to venture higher increased.

This particular Sunday I drove into town. I felt an impatience as I drove the nine miles into Mena. It wasn't the fifteen-miles-an-hour speed that made me impatient, but knowing I would soon be able to climb the steeper grades.

I stopped at my friend's house. He had a garage of sorts there. I had the sprockets geared down so I could go up the steeper grades I yearned to travel. The altered sprockets only allowed the car to travel three to five miles per hour instead of fifteen, but I was happy. The car had extra pull, the pull needed to climb the steeper grades.

It was a beautiful afternoon. As I climbed up the grades I felt like a conqueror. I would stop on top of each mountain and look down onto green hills and thick, dense woods, the bright afternoon sun playing shadow-tricks with the tall pines. It was glorious!

On my way back to the ranch I daydreamed about the color code to the resistor electronics course I was taking, and I forgot to turn the corner that would bring me back to the ranch.

How long I drove I don't remember, but I ended up on a logger's trail where I couldn't turn around. The road was very narrow, and for the first time I regretted not having a reverse gear.

All of a sudden I was going straight up. At times I thought the contraption I created would tip backwards, the grades were so steep, but the car kept crawling right on up, and at times the road seemed to meet the sky.

I thought: *There must be someplace to turn around.* I kept on going.

Soon I was up on top of another mountain and heading down the other side. My ordinary bicycle wheels didn't lend themselves to the stronger braking action needed. My brakes started to smoke, and I was going around the turns much too fast.

All of a sudden I came around a turn and saw a large rattlesnake sunning himself in the road. I had no choice and ran right over him with my front wheel, going so fast it didn't even hurt him. He just jumped a little. I bounced around like a rubber ball, but I was able to bring the car under control. Looking back, I saw the snake lazily crawl off the road into some rocks and brush.

The car sped down around the next turn, and the brakes

refused to hold at all. I wanted adventure, and I was sure getting it!

After much struggling with the steering bar, I was able to straighten the car out. The road leveled off, and the car came to a stop.

After the brakes cooled, I started the car up, pressed the gas lever, and took off again, hoping to find a place to turn around.

It was about four-thirty, and I knew it would be dark soon after six. All I could do was keep on going. I had no headlights, and I prayed that before evening came I would find a place to turn around. However, this was not to be.

"How many mountains?" I groaned. "How many more mountains must I climb?"

Down another grade the brakes gave out again, and I felt my car would tip and spill me out onto the road.

When I reached the bottom of the grade, there was a stream running across the road. The car sped through the stream, the water rushing over the floorboard.

On the other side of the stream was another grade. It was so steep my front wheel raised up off the ground, but the car kept going on up.

As I came to the top of the grade, the back end of the car swayed. I gave the car more gas and it continued on, swaying and grinding away through the dirt road.

How many more mountains must I climb? I thought as I reached the top of the grade. Then I hit a chuckhole and lost my balance. My hand left the gas pedal and the car stopped. It wouldn't start again because I had a centrifugal belt-driven clutch, and the belt was so hot it burned.

Turning the wheels sharply, I let the car roll back a short distance, hoping to end up across the road. The car rolled back too fast and headed right for an embankment.

Reaching out, I grabbed the left back wheel with my hands.

The car stopped just inches away from the embankment. I peered over the cliff and viewed the earth many feet below. Sitting icicle stiff, I wondered if I should let go of the wheel. I wasn't sure how level the ground beneath me was, and I feared the car would roll over the steep cliff.

So many miles from nowhere and all by myself. I thought I was finished. I knew I couldn't jump out of the car before it plunged downward; it always took me several minutes just to climb into the car in my spastic condition.

"O God!" I cried. "Give me the strength to do something!"

Somehow I felt extra strength pour into me, and I grabbed the brake lever as tightly as I could with one hand. Gradually I let go of the back wheel with the other. The car remained still.

"I dare not shake!" I said to the emptiness around me. I sat for awhile and took deep breaths while I prayed for courage.

Then I looked around. The new belt I would have to put on was in the toolbox back of my seat. As I turned and reached for it, I noticed one of the chains on the wheels had broken. I had only one-wheel power now. I would have to find the missing chain.

Swinging one leg over the side of the car with my hands, I let go of it and it struck the ground. Then I put my weight on it and tried to push the car forward. I fell backward, and my body struck the sidebars of the car.

All of a sudden the car was speeding down the grade. The trees became mingled with rapid views of blue sky as the sunlight blinked danger signals through them.

By the time I got to level ground again my head was on the floorboard, my feet on the seat. The car finally came to a stop.

It took me nearly an hour to straighten myself out. When I did right myself to a sitting position, I saw I had ended up just fifteen feet from the creek I had sped through earlier. I would have drowned in that creek if the car had stopped in it, my head on the floorboard. I thanked God for his deliverance.

My shoulder was cut and bleeding and my head was aching. I looked back to see if I could spot the missing chain. It gleamed as the lowering sun's rays bounced off of it. I would have to crawl back up the grade to get it, and I was so exhausted I decided I would have to wait until morning.

I sat and watched the sun move away to the west, knowing by now I could never make it back to the ranch before dark.

All of a sudden I heard something rustle. A large rattlesnake came crawling out of the ditch across the road. He was coming right for me. Maybe the warmth of my gasoline engine was the attraction—I don't know. I took the sling shot I always carried from around my neck, and reaching down I grabbed some rocks. My first and second shots missed. Inserting another rock, I pulled the band back again and released it. The stone struck the snake's head and he dropped.

"Thank God!" I said more loudly than I needed to, alone on a mountain road with only the chilling twilight air and the thick woods to hear.

I glanced up as I sat shivering and shaking. The bright green mountains I had sped through earlier were now bathed in purple hues as the last rays from the sun left me chilled and desolate. I sat and watched the sun until the moon waxed crescent leaving me in almost total darkness.

Mountains are very cold at night. I thought of my sister's ranch house. My mother and father were visiting us at the time. Were they looking for me? They wouldn't be able to find me.

I started rubbing my arms and hands, trying to make my blood move faster through my veins, but it didn't stop the penetrating night air.

I looked at the black woods around me. Then I heard the baying of coyotes far up in the mountains and I began to shiver. I shook so hard my teeth began grinding together.

"O Lord!" I said, as my body shook my little car, "Give me the courage to face this night."

After a while I settled down some until I heard something rustling in the woods to my left. Out stepped a black bear.

My fright was so great my body began to shake from muscle spasms. My heart pounded in rhythm to my jerking, and my head felt as if it would burst, as the black mass came toward me. I knew I must not call attention to myself, and somehow I was able to control my fear. I sat as still as I possibly could.

The bear seemed to look right at me. I closed my eyes, shaking and bouncing as I awaited my fate, crying: "Save me! O my God, save me!"

Then I heard the bear's paws crunch the dirt and rocks in the road and opened my eyes, viewing his massive hind end as he lumbered on down to the creek and on into the woods.

By this time my whole body was damp—frosted by the cold night air. It seemed the temperature was in the twenties, and I felt I would freeze if I didn't stay awake. But staying awake was the easiest task for me by then.

Suddenly through the tops of the trees I saw the face of my grandfather who had died several years earlier.

"Don't give up, Russell," he said, "Help is on the way."

Everyone wonders, I'm sure, when something like this happens, and they ask what tricks their minds are playing. Tricks? Who can truly say? But as I looked into the kind, beautiful face of my grandfather I became immersed in stillness, and I answered: "I'm not afraid."

Several hours later I heard the drone of a helicopter. Then I saw lights from several cars. My father was in the lead car. I discovered after the rescue I was only a half mile or so from the main highway. The Mena newspaper carried the story.

At times like these one's past can become a deep reservoir ready to fill the dry well of loneliness. And so it was that night at the bottom of the mountain as I waited to be rescued. I recalled my past life, becoming warmer as the seasons of my earlier years paraded before my mind. It seemed as though I heard my mother's voice calling to me from out of the past.

"Russ! Where are you, Russ?"

The voice beckoned me back to the safety of our warm kitchen.

At that time we lived on a dairy farm called The Butterfly Dairy. It was just outside the town of Stanton, Nebraska.

Giant stone pillars protected the entrance to the farm. The grounds were beautiful, for my father loved gardening. A lily pond made of colorful stones with a fountain in the middle also added to the landscape, the birds dipping and darting in and out of the fountain. The lily pond was also the summer home for several handsome goldfish.

The house was a two-story frame with a small stoop at the front. At the back of the farmhouse was a large porch, screened in during the summers, offering many pleasant times as the family took to the large table for meals. But the back porch was now covered with a deep white blanket of snow, and the cows in the fields stepped cautiously atop the crusted snow as they struggled to find the familiar fence. It was 1931. I was seven at the time.

The winter storm had ended, and the earth outside held the weight of the six-foot snow. This was a winter I was not to forget.

The smell of my mother's homemade vegetable soup reached my nostrils as I pushed myself into the large kitchen in the kiddie car my father had built for me. This was the only way I could get around the house then except by crawling or rolling.

My mother smiled at me as I entered. She was a stern woman, rather tall, with straight shoulders and strong hands. She had a determined nature, was outspoken, quick-tempered, and impatient, but she quickly forgave.

My father was stern, but patient and forgiving.

My two older brothers were helping with the cows that night.

Buzz was eleven and Bill was thirteen. Toots, my older sister, was fifteen. She was busily setting the table. My younger brother Pete was three at the time, and my baby sister Snooky was one, both too young for the adventure that awaited us older children the following day.

3 Winter: The White Tunnels

Amid the usual clamor and din of children awakening to a new day I heard my brother Buzz shouting to our brother Bill. "We've had another drifting during the night. Come on! Let's climb out the window again and clear some more of the snow; then we'll build tunnels!"

I crawled and rolled into their room just in time to see them jump out of the upstairs window. After struggling to the window I grabbed the window sill, pulled myself up, and looked out over the white landscape.

Dad was just herding the last of the cows into the barn for the morning milking. I looked at the bleak cottonwood tree at the side of the house. Our tree house was covered with snow. Farther away was my uncle's farm. I longed for the excitement of spring and summer, remembering the good times we always had with our cousins.

I looked down at the snow. Buzz and Bill had leaped into it without a thought. How I longed to feel my body flying through the air.

My mother entered the room. "Come on, Russ. Let's get you downstairs and dressed. Old Smokey, the cookstove, is all stoked up and the kitchen is warm. Your dad will finish the milking, and the hired hands will be anxious for their breakfast. Such a storm this has been! It's the worst I've seen!"

"Buzz and Bill are clearing the rest of the snow near the house," I stammered as she picked me up and carried me downstairs.

After I was dressed, she placed me in my kiddie car. My father had made it well. It had wings at the sides and resembled an airplane. He felt the more I exercised my legs the better off I would be. My grandfather also insisted I use all sorts of tools. He was a doctor and felt my hands should be strong even if my legs were not.

After breakfast I sat by the kitchen window and watched Buzz, Bill, and my sister Toots dig the tunnels under the snow. Red mittens, blue mittens, brown mittens, along with tassels on stocking caps, bobbed and danced before my eyes. Clumps of snow were thrown up and out as the three worked frantically to prepare for an exciting day. They would explore the tunnels and play in them when they were finished.

"Will they take me along?" I thought. I pushed myself away from the window and felt my mother's eyes upon me. She knew I was restless, and her face bore a sad look that I am sure matched my own.

"You'll be going to school in the fall, Russ," she said. "The country schoolteacher down the road told me she would enjoy having you. You'll learn and like it, I know."

This pleased me at first. I would be with my older brothers most of the time. Little Pete was too young for my pleasure. But then I remembered that Mom had been a schoolteacher and wished I could be taught at home by her, remembering how the kids in Stanton stared at me when we went to town.

Mom and Pete went out to the barn, leaving me with my baby sister Snooky. She was sleeping by the large cookstove.

Her hair was light just like all of us. It was later in life we changed like chameleons, hair darkening, bodies stretching out, minds searching as we grew.

Buzz came into the kitchen. "Come on, Russ. We're gonna explore the tunnels and play house!" He pulled me from my kiddie car, hurriedly bundled me up, then dragged me from the warm kitchen.

I was happy to say the least! I would be exploring along with the others.

Toots smiled as we entered the tunnel entrance. "Wait until you see, Russ. There are so many passages. We'll explore them all!"

I crawled along behind the others, thrilled by the beauty of the soft white walls surrounding me.

I crawled past many turns, tired but excited. We had peanut butter sandwiches along, and after a while the three left me in one of the tunnels to rest.

I was eating my sandwich when I heard a soft thump. I was trapped by a mountain of snow. The passage was closed! Frantically I tried to dig my way out, but I became so frightened my muscles would not obey my brain. They became like jelly.

Looking at the white walls made me shiver and shake all the more. They had lost their beauty. They were a prison. I was in a prison and couldn't get out! My body shook all the more as my fear of being buried alive increased.

At times like these our minds can lift us up and out of unpleasant and terrifying situations and we end up forgetting where we are and what we're about.

I thought of the school I would be going to. It was three miles from our farmhouse.

"How will I get there?" I said to the cold whiteness. I liked hearing my voice. It was comforting.

"I can't go to school in a kiddie car! The kids will laugh. They'll laugh at me anyway the way I am."

I closed my eyes, slumped forward and placed my head on my arms.

"Dad will build me a wagon! He would never let me go to school in a kiddie car at my age. Yes! He'll build me a nice wagon, I bet. And the pony! Maybe Buzz will pull me to school behind his pony. He will—I know he will!"

It seemed like hours passed before I heard someone clawing at my prison walls. Then my sister Toots poked her head through the snow, and she was the most beautiful sight I had ever seen in all of my seven years.

"Russ! We thought you had died," she cried. Then she stretched her arms up and broke through the top of the tunnel. A mountain of snow came down and buried me. I was terrified and couldn't breathe.

Outside the tunnel Mom and Dad saw my sister wildly waving and they, along with the hired hands, hurried over to her.

After much frantic digging they reached me, finding me pale, gasping, alive, and grateful.

Drinking hot chocolate from a big mug beside a warm cookstove is one of the extreme delights of life.

4 Spring: The Winds of March—A Con Game

It was a warm day late in March. A few patches of snow lay against the south banks of the road and north along the barn. The wind was up, and I felt the promise of April close to delivery.

The sky was bluer than I remembered it during the whiteness of January and February.

Jacket open—capless—I crawled down the back porch steps and rolled across the yard to where my brothers Buzz and Bill were engaged in the art of making a box kite.

I could make some of the sticks! I loved to whittle.

The small wagon with its scooter wheels which my father had made me stood near the barn where my brothers were busily working with the brown paper and twine. I crawled up to the wagon with its box seat for protection and pulled myself up, flopping into it like a seal.

"Good day for kiting," Bill said. "Plenty of wind!"

"Let me cut some of the sticks," I replied, taking out the pocketknife my grandfather had given me.

Buzz looked at me, and I saw his familiar kind wink. "Come on, kid," he said as he tossed several slats of wood he had taken from the barn into the wagon.

I began whittling, feeling the excitement at hand. Soon the kite would be finished, and it would soar up and out. I worked as fast as I could, envisioning the kite and its movement. What a sight it would be when the determined March wind lifted it up, taking it almost to eternity.

The kite was soon finished and the adventure began. Bill ran across the yard, letting the string out a little at a time, the wind lifting the kite. I sat breathless as I watched the brown paper kite soar up over the trees. Higher and higher it ascended until it became only a dark speck, seeming to almost touch a low cloud speeding by. Movement! It was beautiful.

Bill called to Buzz. "Take the twine for awhile. My hands are all burned up from holding it. That wind is so strong I felt myself being lifted up."

Buzz anxiously grabbed the heavy twine. Soon he too was suffering from the pull and the rope burns. "Can't hold it any longer," he said. "My hands are getting raw!"

I pushed myself over to them. "Here, let's tie the twine to the handle of my wagon."

I took the twine and fastened it securely to the handle. I was at the bottom of an incline next to the road at the front of the house, the incline ending at the fence.

All of a sudden I felt the wagon moving as the wind carried the kite and wagon up the incline. Bill and Buzz screamed with delight.

Bill shouted, "Look at him go. Boy! Look at him go!"

"I'm moving. I'm moving up!" I shouted back. The feeling I experienced was one of complete freedom. I didn't have to struggle. I didn't have to push with my hands. I was being borne along by the March wind.

The clatter and bang of a Model T Ford reached my ears. I looked at the road just in time to see the driver staring at me in complete perplexity. He was so intent upon my strange movement upward that his car left the road and plunged into the ditch.

The wagon reached the fence and stopped.

Buzz and Bill ran over to the car as the old man stepped out.

"What on earth!" the old man shouted. "I was so interested in seein' that wagon goin' up a hill for no reason I ended up in the ditch."

SPRING   31

Buzz laughed. "Sorry, mister. There's a kite up there, and the string is attached to my brother's wagon. We'll help you get your car out. I've got a pony!"

Buzz ran to the barn and returned with his pony. He tied a rope to the back bumper of the car and secured the other end to the saddle horn. After several kicks and prods the pony lunged forward. The car was soon out of the ditch.

The old man reached into the pocket of his overalls and handed Buzz a dollar.

Buzz just stood and stared at him for a moment. He grinned. "Gee, thanks, mister," he said as he waved the dollar bill before us.

After the old man was on his way, Buzz came running up to us. "Look! He gave me a whole dollar. What do ya think of that?"

Now as far as I recollect, Bill looked at Buzz, and they both looked at me. It was a look of study and interest.

The next thing I knew they pulled me down the incline and started me up again. I was thrilled to say the least. This was indeed a marvelous thing.

"We'll be rich!" I heard Buzz say. Bill's comment was to the affirmative.

I must also share the blame for what happened next. We became con men.

Buzz and Bill hid the pony in some bushes across the road and we waited for the next car.

They pulled me back down the incline, and trusting to Mother Nature I was once again placed in motion, the wagon rolling up the incline just as the driver of the second car was close enough to observe the strange phenomenon. He, too, ended up in the ditch. I reached the fence and the wagon stopped.

Buzz and Bill hurried around the bushes and pulled the pony from them. I watched as the pony performed his part of the con. Sure enough the grateful driver handed Buzz and Bill some money. We were in business due to the exciting winds of March that aided and abetted us in our con game of Hide the Pony—Send Russ Back Up.

We were almost ten dollars to the good when Dad discovered what we were up to.

We didn't get to keep the money, and Dad felt I was just as much to blame as Buzz and Bill.

My brothers learned that rope burns weren't nearly as painful as raw bottoms, and I also had a hard time sitting.

March finally left us with our wounds along with the lesson that we must not con our fellowmen.

5 Summer: Fish—Tree—Fun—Storm

The summer of my seventh year arrived. It crept up and out onto the landscape releasing butterflies, bees, and worms, along with a burst of colorful petals as the purple violets, pink bellflowers, and yellow lady's slippers swayed and bent in the hot wind. The cornstalks, nearly knee-high, produced movement also as they rustled in the fields. Blue skies with puffy white clouds added to the movement as the summer stretched out before me.

I was sitting by the lily pond one day, offering cracker crumbs to the goldfish as they poked their glistening heads up through the water, anxious for the white morsels. They would purse their small mouths, grab the crumbs, then dart under, their shiny bodies quick with motion.

I wondered what it would feel like to dart through cool water, my legs and arms in perfect harmony, my body shiny and new as a bright penny.

I became restless, crushed the rest of my crackers into small bits and threw them into the pond, feeling discouraged and alone.

Looking up, my eyes searched out the milk house. It was sturdy. Dad built it out of rocks. He had cemented the rocks together and they were firmly fastened. The bottling house next to it was also of rock. It had a cement roof and was connected to the cow barn where the cows were milked. I clinched my fists. The milk house and the bottling house were strong. I was not! Pity? Yes, I pitied myself, for I hated my twisted body and longed to be like everyone else.

Only a nearby robin heard my deep sigh. He flew away as if

he could not stand my sadness and perched on a branch several feet from me.

I became angry and taking my slingshot from around my neck, I picked one of the colored stones from the pond, pulled the band back and released the stone. I was glad I missed the bird, and I watched him fly off toward the barn.

Looking at the big cottonwood tree, green after winter's stripping, gave me no solace. A tree could change. It could be handsome. I could not!

I heard the laughter of my brothers and sisters as they pulled themselves up into the tree house, aided by an old block and tackle. The contraption my brothers had fashioned had a boxlike seat. By pulling on one end of the rope the seat would move upward, offering entrance to the tree house.

I crawled across the yard as my pity diminished and my interest rose.

Bill spotted me. "Hey, Russ! Want to come up?"

Once again the love of my brothers and sisters lifted me, carrying me into adventure and fun.

"We'll send the box seat down for you," Toots yelled. I watched as she pulled at the rope, the seat slowly moving downward.

It thumped onto the ground. I crawled in and pulled at the rope. Again I felt the elation of movement. I was going up, up to the adventure awaiting me.

Reaching the top, I smiled at their crude costumes. "What are you guys doing up here?" I said with anticipation.

Buzz grinned, his white teeth covered with a thick layer of peanut butter. "We're playing jungle and savages. Want a sandwich?"

I settled myself onto the floor of the tree house and proceeded to make my sandwich, relishing the first bite as I looked out over the treetops where my uncle's farm stood. My cousins looked like ants as they scurried about their yard.

After playing in the tree house, riding up and down in the box seat, and after emptying the jar of peanut butter, we stretched ourselves out for a rest.

The sky had changed and so had I. The earlier storm inside me was gone. I had enjoyed a good afternoon in spite of myself, but the blackness I saw through the trees told me another storm was coming.

"Look at those clouds," I said as I pointed upward, slowly twirling my right forefinger in rhythm to the swirls of black and gray.

Dad hollered from the barn. "Buzz! Bill! Pete! Hurry! Help me get the cows to the barn and shut off the windmill!"

The hired hands were no longer with us. The Depression had left scars on us as it had on many.

First Buzz, then Bill, then Pete hurried down in the box seat, leaving Toots, Snooky, and me to see to our own salvation.

Toots placed Snooky's hands on the rope and told her to hang on tight. There was no time for taking turns in the boxseat. The wind was up and the sturdy old tree swayed.

Snooky wrapped her legs around the rope and Toots helped me into the box seat. Then Toots grabbed hold of it and Snooky began her descent.

When Snooky got to the bottom, Toots loosened her grip. As I went down Snooky arose with a squawl. I bounced onto the ground, and Snooky ended up not quite within reach of the tree house, screaming, legs dangling, helpless.

"Grab both ropes!" I shouted. Toots grabbed the ropes, and I slid out of the box seat. Then Snooky descended once again. The box seat went up. Toots climbed into it and soon we were all safely on the ground.

The wind continued to lash out at the cottonwood as I crawled and rolled toward the house, my sisters ahead of me. Thunder struck my ears as if they were pasted to a kettledrum. Lightning flashed as I continued rolling toward the house.

Just before I reached the porch I looked back and saw hot white lightning strike the cottonwood. The tree exploded before my eyes, falling toward me, but I was far enough away. I sat on the ground in shock watching the tree burn, and a feeling of sadness gripped me. Our tree house was gone, but I took heart in the thought I was alive. At least I had managed to maneuver myself to safety. I could take care of myself in an emergency.

Mom stood on the porch steps, a look on her face I will never forget. I could tell she was proud of me.

"Come on, Russ," she shouted as Toots and Snooky scrambled up onto the porch. "Get in here before you drown!"

Those words may not seem very important, but they were to me. Her voice spelled out: that boy can take pretty good care of himself.

Through that experience I learned several things. I realized I could be helpful in an emergency. I felt I could take care of myself, and I also learned that movement didn't always have to be fast—just accurate. Where I was headed and where I was going seemed to take on more importance. That day I had fallen into the swamp and mire of self-pity, later discovering that by looking up and away from it I could find another kind of movement—a movement toward better things, happiness in enjoying the world around me. Although I questioned this discovery many times later in life, I know it to be a sound one.

The following day Mom and Dad left us at home and went into Stanton on business. It was a hot day, steaming from the storm that had ravaged our farm the day before. The torrent of rain had descended upon the fertile fields and the ditches along the road were filled to near overflowing. We were warned not to get our clothes muddy.

Mud was no problem, because after our cousins came down the road to join us, we all stripped and quickly sought the cool comfort of one of the ditches. I sat in a high spot, muddy water up to my waist. Digging my toes into the soft bank was soothing.

Whenever a car passed by, we would wave and giggle and then slip beneath the muddy water to hide our nakedness.

Later that night we were summoned before the cookstove. Mom and Dad stood lion-like, their eyes ablaze. But in back of the blaze I saw a spark of humor and thanked the Lord for it.

Mom spoke first. "It's a darn good thing you kids didn't ruin your clothes. We can be grateful for that at least!"

Dad shouted: "Shameful! Making a public spectacle of yourselves. Stripping bare and swimming naked as the neighbors drove by. This will not happen again! If it does, I'll buy a cat-o'-nine-tails and strip all the skin from your bones. Now get to bed!"

We scurried out of the kitchen and up the stairs, grateful for a second chance.

Sometimes parents spit out sharp words because of their anxiety over the safety and morality of their children as innocently as a lioness swats her cubs with her paw as she strives to teach them survival—just a slice of the pie of life.

The fall of my seventh year I consumed more slices of the pie of life, and they also helped to sustain me that night I was trapped in the Arkansas mountains as I sat half-frozen and alone, remembering my three years at the country school.

6 Fall: School—Outhouse—Pillsbury Panties—Redhead

September arrived, hot and humid, and I sought the comfort of the lily pond. The tree house was no more. I could never be on top of the world again.

As I plunged my fist into the cool water of the pond, my favorite goldfish swam around it as if he were playing Here We Go 'Round the Mulberry Bush. I remembered how Buzz, Bill, and Toots walked around the big bush in our yard when they were younger, singing the familiar verses that accompanied the old nursery game.

I drew my hand from the water and slowly raised it. I was so slow at everything. I couldn't walk around a mulberry bush, I would have to crawl. Once again I became immersed in self-pity, wishing I were a mulberry bush. I would be more important as a bush. Birds could nest in my branches and kids could play around me. I wouldn't ever be lonesome.

"Mulberry bushes are pretty," I said as I looked at my reflection in the pond. "Mulberry bushes let you play games of hide and seek, or just plain hide!"

I thought about the country school. Monday I would be in that school, the kids staring and making fun of me like they did in Stanton. On my trips into town with Mom and Dad the kids always pointed and laughed, their parents giving me looks of pity combined with ones of horror as they nudged, slapped, or shoved their little ones away from me.

At the school I would be in close contact with my classmates. This confinement would last from Mondays through Fridays, my only escape being Saturdays and Sundays.

The mulberry bush indeed. Mondays I would not be able to

watch Mom wash our clothes, feeling the comfort of her nearness. Tuesdays I would miss watching her determined strokes with the flatiron as she smoothed out the wrinkled clothes. And so on and on through Fridays. I would be separated from the familiar household tasks of my mother as I struggled in my kiddie car to keep up with her movements, being comforted by her closeness.

I heard the back door slam and looked up. Mom, her apron covering her Sunday dress, walked down the steps and came over to me.

She stood, her hands on her hips, a smile on her face, but her blue eyes held a knowing expression. How did she know when I was sad? How did she always know?

She sat on the big rock beside the pool and folded her hands as if in prayer. Her fingers became spotted with white as they pressed against each other.

"The chicken is all batter-dipped and ready to fry when we get back from church, Russ. We're having your favorite dessert—chocolate pie. Now look at you!" she scolded. "You've gone and gotten your nice white shirt sleeve wet. What's wrong? You've been as restless as Caesar, our bull. It's the school, isn't it? Well, isn't it?"

"I don't want to go, Mom," I cried, as my mind forced my right hand to the task of wringing out the wet sleeve of my shirt.

"Now Russ, this is something you must do. You must get an education," she continued. "You know Miss Daniel, your teacher. She's been here for supper and talked with you. She told you everything would work out fine. You must learn to trust people more. You will go to school!

"Anyway, think of the fun you'll have when Buzz pulls you along behind his pony in your wagon. You're a very lucky boy. Now come on," she said, as she pushed herself up from the rock. "I don't want to hear any more nonsense from you. Hurry on now. We don't want to be late for church."

She left me well-scolded and with a feeling of finality. There was no getting out of it; I was going to school! I knew this as surely as I knew our bull, Caesar, would attend to his duty Monday morning when my uncle brought his cow over to be serviced.

Monday morning arrived, as I knew it would. Holding back the dawn of a new day along with one's movement through it can never be accomplished, but if it had been possible I would have especially prolonged the dark night before as I lay beside my little brother Pete. Did he too know when I was sad? So young—only three?

His familiar foot pushed at mine under the sheet. "Don't go to school, Russ." He began to cry.

I spasmed my hand out and found his tiny one. "I want to go to school!" I shouted at him. "I want to learn things. I'm gonna learn to write. I'll write you stories and read to you. Stop cryin'," I said, as my voice softened.

"Gee, that's fun," he giggled as he snuggled closer to me. "Write ponies—I like ponies!"

"OK, I'll write ponies," I answered. "Now get to sleep."

I'll never forget the feel of his tiny hand as he reached up and patted my face. Soon I heard his soft breathing.

I pushed myself up and looked out of the window. Shadows fell across the yard as the big yellow moon moved from behind a cloud, and I heard the baying of the coyotes.

I remembered what the preacher had said at church. "If God be for us, who can be against us?" I cherished this thought most of the night as I lay thinking about the school, watching the moon and stars pop in and out of the clouds. Exhausted, but calm, I fell asleep.

It seemed like only minutes passed until Buzz and Bill rushed into the room. Bill pulled the sheet off.

"Come on, lazybones! We'll be late for school," he shouted as he picked Pete up and moved him to the foot of the bed.

Little Petiesweet crawled up into a ball, not yet ready to face his day, and, to say the least, I wasn't either.

Buzz and Bill pulled me from the bed. They placed me on the floor and hurried out of the room.

Buzz looked back at me. "Hurry up, kid. I'll give you a ride you won't forget!"

After a hurried breakfast, Buzz tied a rope to the handle of my wagon. He then tied the other end of the rope to his saddle horn, mounted, gave the pony a good prod, and we were off and running.

Mom shouted: "Be careful now! Take care of him, Buzz."

My wagon wheels resisted the sharp turn as the pony bounded out the gate. The box seat my dad had built for my protection was of little use, and I spilled out onto the ground, box seat and all. I rolled and bounced like a tumble-weed, collecting dust in my mouth, my eyes, and on my newly patched hand-me-down knickers. One of the patches at the knee left its finely stitched position my mother had placed it in, and I felt the sharp pain as a rock tore at my flesh. I trembled and shook from the unfortunate upset.

As I tried to right myself to a sitting position, clutching and clawing for balance, I heard Mom shout: "Now see what you've done! Buzz, if you ever do anything like that again while you're in charge of your brother I'll smack you good!"

She knelt down and picked me up. I felt her body sway, the muscles in her arms quivering under the strain.

Dad took the reins from Buzz and brought them down sharply onto Buzz's legs. "You mind what you're told!" Dad said between clenched teeth.

Then he noticed my skinned knee, and he took me from my mother's arms. "Buzz, when you get to the school you be sure and wash off his knee at the pump." He placed me back into the box seat and set it in the wagon. "Now get going before you're late."

I felt bad. I was ashamed. I was always trouble somehow. I felt sorry for myself and my family.

My shame and self-pity were short-lived though as Buzz again prodded the pony. The pony bolted out onto the road, the wagon bouncing along behind. Buzz pulled back on the reins and the pony settled down into a trot.

I clutched the side of the box seat, my raw knee stinging, but I felt an excitement as the wagon bounced over ruts and chuck holes.

As we passed one of the farms, another boy on a pony came out onto the road. He smiled at Buzz. I saw the challenge in his eyes.

Buzz immediately took up that challenge, and we were off and running again, the wagon bouncing up and down, my bottom kneading the old leather cushion placed there for my comfort.

When we got to the school, I looked back. Buzz was three lengths ahead of his friend. We had won the race!

My brother Bill, who had left earlier, was standing in the schoolhouse yard.

"Good boy!" he shouted. Then he came running up to us. "Ya beat old Highpockets again!"

"We sure did," I stammered with pleasure.

After a few quick, stinging splashes of cold water from the pump, my raw knee, which I had forgotten about, looked more presentable.

My brothers lifted the box seat from the wagon and carried me to the school steps just as Buzz's friend Highpockets blocked them.

"Think you're somethin', don't ya?" he said, a half-grin on his face.

"Come on," Buzz complained. "This thing is heavy."

Highpockets kicked at the dirt with his bare feet and moved aside, giving me a devilish grin.

Before I knew it the box seat was shoved onto the chair attached to my desk. The desk had been reconstructed to make room.

Buzz and Bill took their places just as Miss Daniel entered the room.

She walked to the front of the room. I'll never forget her warm smile as she turned and looked at me. I believe I fell in love with her at that moment.

I was at the front of the room and this made it easier for me. I only heard the snickers of the other children. I didn't have to look into their faces; Miss Daniel had seen to that. How I loved her!

The time went by fast as I listened to her read about the beginning of our country. The struggle for freedom excited me. I pretended I was Paul Revere, and I could almost see myself riding bravely through the cobblestone streets of Boston.

The question and answer period began. Buzz had warned me about it, and I had promised to help him. He hated to stand and recite.

Buzz looked over and shot me the familiar signal. The roll of his eyes set me into motion, and I raised my hand.

"Yes, Russell?" Miss Daniel said impatiently.

I froze! How could I tell her out loud I wanted to go to the outhouse? I swallowed hard, my vocal chords resisting the instructions from my brain.

She saved me. "Buzz, take your brother outside please."

Buzz jumped from his seat, picked me and the box seat up like we were mere feathers, and carried us out of the school.

"You did real good, kid," he said as he carried me down the steps to the outhouse.

When we returned, our classmates were busily writing. Buzz had won another victory. Buzz winked at me, and I was proud I had helped even though I felt a slight prick from Mr. Conscience.

After recess and some more goading between Buzz, Bill, and

Highpockets, my brothers picked me up and carried me back to the schoolhouse steps.

Now Buzz and Bill must take the blame for what happened next. Accident? Perhaps.

In front of me was a mass of flaming red hair and a full skirt sprinkled with little yellow flowers. My brothers tipped the box seat backward, and my feet lifted the girl's skirt up. I stared at the Pillsbury label on the seat of her pants.

Buzz and Bill laughed as they viewed the familiar label which represented the increasing poverty that plagued the country.

"Flour sack underwear?" Bill said, amazed at the sight of the label.

The girl swirled around and glared at us, and I fell in love for the second time that day. Her blue eyes flashed. She tossed her flaming mane back like a determined filly, giving the box seat a kick, the front of her underpants free of the telltale label.

"Think you're smart!" she scolded. "Well! Elsie Robins and Agatha Montgomery have flour sack pants, too! They even have flour sack undershirts! You think you're smart!"

She was beautiful. She had smiled at me. I was truly in love.

During the three years I spent at that school, my Pillsbury girl sat and played checkers with me or we talked when the weather was too cold for me to be taken out for recess. She helped me to learn true compassion.

When school was dismissed that first day, Buzz and Bill were delayed somewhat, a slight penance for their misbehavior.

I was sitting in the wagon near Buzz's pony when all of a sudden Highpockets, the boy who had lost the early morning race with Buzz, came charging at me, his pony in full gallop. He relaxed his reins, and the pony jumped over my head barely clearing it with its hooves.

Buzz and Bill were coming down the schoolhouse steps. Buzz rushed over to Highpockets and pulled him from his pony then shoved him to the ground and began delivering his blows, shouting: "If you ever come near our brother again, I'll make mincemeat out of ya!"

Bill checked me over carefully, and I felt another kind of love that day—a kinship love that can only be experienced between brothers and sisters at certain given times. My brothers were my protectors from then on.

As I lay next to little Pete that night he asked: "You like school, Russ? Did ya write ponies?"

"No ponies yet, Petiesweet," I answered as I thought about everything that happened to me throughout the day. My foot finally reached his and I said, "It will be a long time before I can write ponies, but I think I like school—I think so."

The following day the snickering of the other children had dwindled. Only a few of them nudged each other as I entered the schoolhouse. I was very happy to see they had lost interest in me.

Miss Daniel changed somewhat toward me though. I couldn't make my pencil move in the right direction. I was nervous, and my mind and hands just wouldn't work together. Disgusted, I snapped the pencil in half.

Miss Daniel looked up from her desk. "Russell, we do not break pencils or let go of our emotions in the schoolroom."

She left her desk and came up to me. "Here," she said as she handed me another pencil. "These cost a nickel. Now try again. You will learn to write along with the others!"

Again I tried, and the boy sitting next to me laughed as my fingers struggled to make marks on the paper.

I broke the second pencil and threw the pieces onto the floor, placed my head on my arms, and hid my tears.

I felt the sharp pain as Miss Daniel's ruler came down across my knuckles. I looked up at her defiantly.

"All right, Russell Schultze, you will stay after school for breaking your pencil again. I will help you with your writing then," she said, a determined look on her face.

She glared at the boy next to me. "You will stay after school also. And you will write the letters ABC ten times each. This punishment is to help you to learn that to laugh at someone less fortunate than yourself is wrong. Buzz and Bill Schultze learned that lesson yesterday. Now everyone get to work!"

After handing me another pencil, she went to her desk. I struggled through the day feeling Petiesweet would never get his pony stories.

After three years at the country school I wrote several stories for little Pete. I cannot write very well to this day, but at least I can write. Miss Daniel's determination won me this satisfaction, and because of her experiences with me she decided to further her education and learn more about teaching the handicapped. In later years I looked back and realized that if I hadn't been handicapped perhaps Miss Daniels wouldn't have gone into special teaching skills which help others like myself.

The Depression finally took our farm, and we moved just outside Stanton into a rented house with just enough of our farm stock left to continue in the dairy business while Dad searched for extra employment. He had been a school principal at one time, and his good record helped. He became the county clerk.

I missed the lily pond and the many cows, the green fields, and the movement of the old windmill.

It was at this time my parents felt the orthopedic hospital at Lincoln, Nebraska, would be able to help me. The hospital at Lincoln offered hope. I was ten when my parents drove me into Lincoln and left me there for treatment.

Those three years at the hospital became a nightmare as my muscles fought the cast covering most of my body. It was then that I changed, becoming swept into another world, a world I never again want to enter, a world of bleak shadows and shapes, a world of little crystalline people, a world of horror!

7 The Great Impasse: A Mountain of Plaster

It was one of the hottest days I can ever remember. As I lay in bed the night before the trip to the orthopedic hospital at Lincoln, Nebraska, the August heat crept through the window screen.

I struggled to pull down the shade. Sinking back onto the bed, I lay gasping as the sweat trickled over my body, shivering in spite of the heat, knowing that after the journey to Lincoln I would no longer be in the care of my parents.

I remembered the red wagon I had seen in the store that morning. It had headlights and balloon tires, and I decided I would save up my allowance and buy it someday.

This thought soon left me, and I wondered what the hospital would be like. I had never seen one. Some of the stories I picked up earlier from visiting grown-ups were heartening—most were not. I remembered hearing about the suffering that went on in them and I was afraid.

Then I remembered the ancient words in the Bible, words my mind stored up because of the church attendances with my parents and I thought: A mustard seed! A mustard seed can help you. If you have the faith of a mustard seed you can move mountains!

Taking heart from this thought, I prayed: "God, I don't understand all of this faith yet, but please give me the faith of a mustard seed."

Morning arrived, and after the bustle and the parting tears of my brothers and sisters, Mom and Dad nervously stuffed me into the car and we were off for Lincoln.

The trip was exhausting, the road dusty, the hot August sun

blistering the black paint on our old Model A Ford.

After three tire changes and much spouting and steaming, we reached Lincoln.

We spent the night at my Uncle Red's house. He was very kind to me, and Aunt Regina saw that I was comfortable.

The next morning my parents took me to the hospital.

As the wheelchair, pushed by a sanitary-looking nurse, neared the car, I began to shake. Dad placed his twitching son into the hospital chair, and the nurse wheeled me up the ramp and into the lobby.

There were so many wheelchairs we almost had a traffic jam as the nurse pushed me around a corner.

"This won't be so bad," I thought. "There are many like me. I'll meet others. I'll make friends. We'll talk and have nice times together." I bit my lip and tried to control my shaking body.

After my parents answered many questions at the main desk, the nurse busily writing my history, I was taken to one of the wards. Mom and Dad anxiously trotted along beside me as the nurse reassured them.

"Your son will be well taken care of. They are doing wonders these days. Many have walked out of here."

I liked hearing her words. Maybe—maybe I would walk someday. Maybe my body wouldn't jerk. This gave me hope. The mustard seed thought from the night before became more than just a thought. I felt it was a means by which I could turn hope into reality if I could muster up enough faith. But as the nurse pushed me through the doors of the ward, I saw many bodies covered by mountainous white plaster casts and shuddered, my nervousness making my muscles jump all the more. I shook so hard my body jerked in every direction.

One smile, one beautiful smile helped me. A little tow-headed boy lay in his bed. His legs were spread out and slightly bent inside two casts. He looked like a frog.

THE GREAT IMPASSE

I smiled at him as my jumping muscles fought my brain. "Will they do that to me?" I wondered. "Well, if he can stand it, I can. He must be six or seven. He reminds me of Petiesweet."

After a briefing from Mom and Dad as to how I was to conduct myself, they left, Mom saying, "Be a good boy now." Dad's good-bye was curt. "You do as you're told."

"They don't care anything about me," I thought. "They just don't care!" Then I remembered the looks on their faces. They cared! I took comfort from their sad and worried expressions.

After the nurses pinned me beneath the sheet in order to stop me from bouncing out of the bed, salty rivulets reached my lips, and I licked at my sadness.

I glanced over at the tow-headed little frog and he smiled again, his brown-velvet eyes searching my watery blue ones. I remembered the mustard seed again and throught: "He's got one of them. He must have a mustard seed to put up with that white mountain covering him."

"How-long-have-you-been-here?" I asked, my voice sounding like a damaged Caruso record.

"I dunno," he answered as he tossed his coloring book over to me. "Wanna see?"

My shaking hands clutched the book, and I looked at the cover. Boys and girls were dancing around a Maypole. Ribbons of pink, yellow, blue, green, red, and orange were twisted from the top almost to the bottom of the pole. The picture book was so colorful it lifted my spirits. I opened the cover. Soft delicate strokes from several crayons had turned the outlined figures of a boy and his dog fishing into a masterpiece as far as I was concerned. I thought of the lily pond in our yard at The Butterfly Dairy, the goldfish dipping and diving, free to swim and play beneath the water.

"We-had-a-big-lily-pond-on-our-farm-with-goldfish-in-it," my staccato voice announced.

"I never had a goldfish. I like fish." He grinned.

The doctor came into the room followed by an army of nurses with strange looking caps that gave them a caricatured appearance. I became more upset as they worked their way over to me.

The doctor looked at the little frog. "Well now," he said as he rapped on one of the little frog's casts. "How are you today, Jimmy?"

"Fine! Want to see my picture book? He's got it."

"I sure do, Jimmy," the doctor answered. "You're a real artist. What have you colored today? Let's take a look."

The doctor then turned to me and held out his hand. I spasmed my arm out and handed him the picture book, his eyes watching my erratic performance.

He smiled. "When I finish seeing what Jimmy has been up to, I'll check you over and see what's to be done."

A curtain was drawn around me by one of the nurses and the doctor stepped inside. I saw the frown on his face as he stared at my thin body and twisted legs. He nodded to the nurse and left. The nurse helped me into a white gown, pinned the sheet over me, and left also. I was cut off from little Jimmy for the rest of the night, but his soft babbling and happy chuckling helped calm me and I slept.

After a week of bloodletting, as the nurses and interns helped themselves to whatever they needed, I was taken to a large room that smelled of wet plaster. The odor sickened me.

I began to shake as one of the nurses placed a mask over my face telling me to take deep breaths.

When I awoke I was back in my bed, legs aching, body rigid. I shuddered as I looked down and saw the cast from my armpits to my ankles, and I began to cry.

"Gee! You got a bigger one!" a voice said. I looked over and the little frog was smiling, a look of admiration in his eyes.

Little Jimmy and I did very well for several months. We kept each other company, and he always seemed to lift my spirits.

THE GREAT IMPASSE

I cried the day he left, but I was happy for him. His cast was gone, and his problem was solved.

"Bye, Russ," he grinned. "You'll look nice, too. Thanks for the goldfish."

Little Jimmy picked up his goldfish bowl, walked to the door, then turned. "I'm gonna get a bicycle. Yes sir, a red bicycle!"

After he left I lay desolate. Life wouldn't be the same without him. He had taken the place of Petiesweet in many ways.

Mom and Dad came to see me the next day with good news. Mom smiled. "Russ, we have a surprise for you. You remember that red wagon you saw in the store window the day before we left for Lincoln? Well, your brothers and sisters saved up their money and bought it for you. It's at home waiting." Mom's face lit up with a satisfied grin. "What do you think of that?"

I tried to raise up, I was so excited. "The one with the headlights? The one with the balloon tires?"

"That's the one," Dad said proudly. "Now you get well, and when you come home, it's all yours."

This news brightened my outlook, and I lay anxious for the day when I could leave the hospital. The thought of the shiny new wagon waiting for me made my stay more bearable.

As the months wore on, many patients came and went. I tried to comfort them as the little frog had done, even relating my remembrance of the mustard seed, telling them that Jesus would help it grow, praying mine would grow, too.

But as time passed I became very uncomfortable. My spastic muscles had fought every inch of the cast and soon the pain was unbearable. I developed pressure-ulcers. Blood ran out of my cast onto my toes and out of the opening at my crotch. The odor from the blood and urine was sickening. I screamed for more narcotics, praying for escape from the pain and vomitus odor.

One day I awoke from my dream world the drugs had placed me in and felt activity underneath my cast. It was unbelievable, but something was crawling all over me.

"What is it?" I shouted, my body turning to ice as the crawling, sucking feeling spread over me.

"They're just maggots," the nurse said. "They will eat up the dead flesh and help heal your pressure-ulcers."

I screamed as the carnivorous larvae from dipterous insects continued feeding on my raw flesh, remembering the maggots out by the barn as they finished off a dead field mouse the cats had killed and tired of. I shuddered and couldn't stop screaming.

The nurse plunged a needle into my arm. Soon my screams were softer and softer. Faint voices reached my ears. The room became dim—blurred. Then I was swept into a vortex of dull noises and darkness and on into nothing.

After that horrible afternoon I didn't seem to want to remember anything. Visits from my parents and aunt and uncle soon drifted away, and they became forgotten people as I slept, my mind buried beneath heavy drugs. Every waking minute I screamed for more of the drugs as the painful ulcers and the memories of the maggots plagued me.

Often I was put into a large bathroom by myself so as not to disturb the other patients. The drugs were administered as promptly as was the hospital custom.

I was living in two worlds now, one of blissful sleep and one of horror and pain.

One day between one world and the other my mother came to visit me. "Russell," she cried, her face white. "I could hear you screaming a block away!"

Soon she became a floating entity before my eyes. Her voice was barely audible, and I drifted off again into the dark world of narcotics.

My grandfather, Dr. Edgar Sears, from Decatur, Nebraska, visited me several times during those years. I loved him dearly.

THE GREAT IMPASSE

One day he came with my mother and father and saw the state I was in. He scowled. "You must take Russ out of here. It's about time you stopped worrying about his walking. It's about time he made something of himself. Look at him! He won't live if you don't take him home."

My mother, trusting to the wise counsel of her father, insisted I go home.

The cast was removed after those three years of suffering, and I was nothing but raw meat. My brain suffered also. The drugs had left me with a brain no better than a turnip—a shriveled one at that. It could no longer command my body as it had once struggled to do.

I screamed when the air hit my rawness. Then I was submerged into a tub of warm water, and this helped some. The nurse left me to see about another patient. The shot I had received minutes before began to work. My body wouldn't allow me the thrust needed, and I slipped beneath the water, unable to move. I lay holding my breath.

"I'll drown!" I thought. I lay there staring through my watery grave. "The mustard seed—the mustard seed!" my shriveled mind signaled, and I continued holding my breath until I felt I could hold it no longer. I struggled to remember the words I had heard at church. "Faith—mustard seed! Mountains—move mountains! Dear Jesus!"

Somehow I found enough strength to continue without air, feeling I was floating, my head reeling, and I thought my chest would burst.

Then above the still water I saw a troubled face. Hands clawed at me, and I was lifted from the tub. I gasped for air.

"Are you all right?" the nurse cried, her eyes glistening with tears.

Between gasps of freedom I answered, "I think so. I guess so!" I was like a slippery eel by then. I had no control of my body at all, but I realized how precious life was.

Much later, after I was home, fighting off the drug habit I acquired in the hospital, I learned the doctors had told my parents I would not live but a few months, but I discovered that faith and determination make a powerful antidote for death.

8 The Road Back: A Psychogenic Journey

After a few weeks, as my body sores continued to heal, Mom and Dad took me from the hospital. I had braces from my armpits down to my toes, my shoes were molded onto the bottom of the braces. Robot-stiff they placed me into the car. It was early morning.

As we traveled home, the road and sky sped by me. I wanted to scream. My nerves seemed to rip; my muscles quivered like a wounded animal in a trap. The braces tightened against me, and I shuddered. My flesh strained against metal.

I screamed, and my father almost ran us into a ditch.

He reached back and slapped me. It wasn't a hard slap. He just wanted to calm me down.

Mom was in the backseat with me. She freed me from my braces in order to give me more movement, thinking this would help my nervousness.

Nothing helped, and I twisted and turned until my nerves were on fire. Another scream escaped from me.

By now my parents realized I was in need of more narcotics. They had been told I was an addict. "Hang on, Russ," Mom cried. "Hang on, Son!" she begged, as I thrashed and babbled.

All of a sudden my mind began to play tricks on me. I cringed as the line of cars coming at us on the other side of the road came nearer. As each car reached us it split before my eyes and rushed past on both sides of the road. My eyes couldn't focus even though I blinked them several times. The telephone poles became people. As we passed by they grinned at me, their eyes hollow—empty.

Mom gave me some aspirins, but they didn't help. Dad finally stopped the car and got out to check the tires. We had stopped near a fence where some cows stood. The cow's faces took on the faces of some of the patients and nurses I had seen at the hospital. The trip home was a nightmare of distorted faces and shiny, split automobiles.

When we entered the living room, I saw my red wagon. One headlight was smashed and one of the balloon tires was flat. I felt I was seeing things again until Dad put his arm on my shoulder, saying: "Pete had an accident the other day. Don't worry, Son, we'll get the wagon fixed."

I had waited for two years for a shiny red wagon. It was broken and so was I. I hated my brother Pete that night.

The following day Mom and Dad took me to the doctor in Stanton and explained to him I was addicted to drugs. He gave Mom some weaker ones for me to take in order to bring me down slowly.

They didn't help, and I couldn't sleep. I had lived in my dream world too long. I wasn't even able to feed myself, my body was so out of control, my brain was too damaged to make the necessary commands. A year passed and still I suffered from the want for stronger drugs, sometimes crawling up into a ball as I screamed for relief. But as time passed my deep desire lessened and my strength returned. Mom's prayers and determination saw to that. I'm sure that family prayers, along with my own, were responsible for my deliverance from the drugs.

One day Dad brought home a radio. It was an old Philco with a rounded wooden top. Often my brothers took me from my bed and carried me into the living room. We would all sit around and listen to the programs. One special program presented at night always left Pete hiding under a chair and Buzz behind it. The program, *I Love a Mystery*, was too much for us, but my brother Bill teased and coaxed us out of our fears, and we always enjoyed that program with its thrills and chills.

The last hallucination I remember having happened one day

as I was listening to "Ma Perkins," a daytime serial. I was lying in my bed. I looked at the radio and suddenly the voices sounded like the voices of some of the nurses and patients at the hospital. Out popped little crystalline figures—very transparent—about two inches high. They came in hordes, marching out of the radio and moving all around the room. They crawled over the furniture and curtains. Closer and closer they came, marching up the walls, and onto my bed. As the glass army reached me I screamed.

Mom came running into the room and snapped off the radio. The figures disappeared.

"Too much radio," Mom said in disgust. "Some of those programs are ruining children. The broadcasters should watch what they put on the air!"

She covered my quivering body, then leaned down and kissed my cheek. "You settle down now and get some rest. Lunch will be ready soon."

I didn't tell her what I had experienced. I didn't want to worry her, and I prayed the strange sights I had seen would be removed forever. They ended that day.

Mom was still feeding me at the time. But that day she presented me with quite a problem. She entered my room, pulling my red wagon behind her with my lunch neatly placed inside it. With a determined look she pushed the wagon sideways beside my bed. Then she picked me up and flipped me over onto my stomach. I stared at the plate of food as she patted me firmly on the back.

"Now Russ, you must learn to feed yourself. Lean over there and pick up your spoon. I'll not give you one bite! You must learn to feed yourself again. No more until supper time either!" She left the room.

I forced my hand down and clumsily clutched the spoon. My hand shook, and I spilled the first spoonful into the bottom of the wagon. I cried; I had dirtied it.

I wiped my tears, angry at my mother, and disgusted with myself. As I tried again my face slipped into the mashed potatoes. I sputtered and gasped but managed to lift my face out of the warm white mass. More tears ran onto the plate and mixed with the red juice from the beets.

Mom stuck to her decision though and forbade anyone to help me. She was determined I would learn to feed myself once again. I hated meals, and I fought to keep my faith in myself and the Lord.

Sometimes my sister Toots would sneak up, take the spoon, and offer me several bites of food, then dash out of the room like a child expecting to be caught at the cookie jar. I enjoyed the smirking satisfaction I felt when Mom would come in and say: "My, Russ, you're doing better. I knew you could do it!"

My coordination improved in spite of the grudge against my mother, and one day when I saw the look of pride in her eyes after she had witnessed weeks of trial and error and a very messy wagon, I realized her sternness and determination had given me the opportunity to gain back my self-respect. My brain had once again taken possession of my body. My body grew stronger each day, and my spirit to continue on also returned.

Summer came, and little Pete went to visit my uncle and aunt in Lincoln. My little cousin traded places with him for awhile. She was around two and a half then. I would lie on the floor and listen to the radio, and many times she toddled over to me and sat on my head. Not yet being potty trained, sometimes she let loose, and my face would be wet. This acid action most certainly added to my determination to make my brain and hands work as they once had.

To say the least, I was pleased when she went home and Pete came back to us. I'll never forget that day. He came home with a miracle. Uncle Red had taught him how to play chess and had bought him a chess set.

THE ROAD BACK

Pete opened out the chessboard that evening and placed the two armies on it.

"This is the way it goes, Russ," he said as he made the first move. "The little men in front go forward. The queen here can go anyplace quick. Kings get only one move at a time, knights hop around like this, and bishops go this way. Then these rooks move up and down and across."

I was fascinated as he slowly moved the little wooden figures around the board. After my mind soaked up the procedure, we began. Pete beat me badly.

I became so fascinated with the game that I sat for hours and manipulated both the black and white chessmen. In a few weeks Pete gave up. He could beat me no longer. He didn't seem to mind though as he sat and watched me checkmate the whole family. He was proud and so was I. I had discovered something I could really do well because of Pete sharing his miracle game with me.

I studied many chess books after that. I was free of the drug habit, and I thanked God. Maybe I couldn't walk, and maybe I never would, but I could use my mind and this I did.

In 1939 we moved into Stanton proper and rented a house on a hill. I was fifteen, and I didn't have much chance to meet people. Pete and Snooky continued their schooling at the grade school. Bill and Toots had moved to Illinois and were working in the Quad Cities. They were both married at this time, and Buzz had joined the CCC camp which was created by President Roosevelt to put young men to work for the government. Mom, Dad, Pete, Snooky, and myself were left at home. I was lonely with almost half of my family gone.

One day there was a special program at the school. I was allowed to go. Pete pulled me there in my wagon.

We arrived at the school, and after much maneuvering Pete pulled me into the schoolroom.

I was surrounded by children again. They stared as children usually did, but the teacher took me to the front of the room and the program began.

There was a woman with trained birds. It was quite a show. One little green parakeet could do almost anything. I fell in love with him.

After the show the woman came up to me. She handed me the parakeet, cage and all. "I want you to have him," she said.

I couldn't believe my ears. I was thrilled and thanked her. "I'll-take-good-care-of-him—real-good-care," I stammered, excited over the precious gift.

She smiled down at me. "I'm sure you will," she said, as she turned and walked back to collect her other pets.

Pete pulled me back home, and when we entered the kitchen Mom was at the cookstove. She turned around.

"What on earth have you there?" she questioned.

"A bird, Mom," I answered as I pulled the cover from the cage. "Isn't he beautiful?"

"I will declare, Russ. If I sent you to a circus, you'd come home with an elephant," she scolded, as she stood waving the large wooden spoon at me.

She wasn't smiling, and I was worried.

"Oh, well," she finally added, "hurry and get washed up for supper. We must eat early tonight. Your father has to be back at the courthouse. There's a special meeting. Sometimes I wish he wasn't the county clerk. It keeps him away from the house too much. He's a dairy farmer, not a politician. Hurry on now!"

I quickly obeyed, hoping she wouldn't later reject my pet.

As the weeks passed a tutor was found for me. I worried about this, wondering what she would be like. Would she be as nice as Miss Daniel at the country school?

The day she came little Buddy, my parakeet, left my shoulder and flew to hers. I thought, "If he likes her, I like her." She was pleasant and we got along well.

Summer arrived, and I became restless and lonely. Pete and Snooky would play outdoors with the other children until supper time. I took my pleasure with little Buddy. He was truly free and could fly anyplace in the house. I liked watching him drink from the dripping faucet in the kitchen. There was no fountain for me. I thought of the lily pond again and the fountain there. How I longed to return to my earlier days on the farm with my brothers and sisters.

Pete came running into the house one day and announced that the WPA had just opened a recreation center in Stanton. I persuaded him to push me down there. He did, and a whole new world opened up for me that summer.

Once inside the hall a man came up to me. "I'm Max Patch," he said. "What would you like to do?"

I stammered, "Play—play chess."

"Well, that can be arranged." He looked at Pete. "What do you like to do?"

Pete bashfully pounded his fist into his baseball glove and turned. "I like to play outside!"

After Pete's quick exit, Max Patch motioned to one of the boys and soon I was engaged in a chess match.

Max watched, and after I won he sat down opposite me and I won again. However, I didn't win all of the matches by a long shot. Max was quite a challenge.

What a summer I had. Max taught me how to make knick-knack shelves and corner shelves. He also urged me to make jewelry along with the others. I enjoyed being with them. They seemed to accept a sandy-haired cripple in a red wagon because of his ability to play chess and make things, and I was happy.

One day Max asked: "How would you like to make a bow? I'm sure you can do it. Your hands are strong, and when we finish our bows I'll take you out and we'll have target practice."

This was another challenge, and I was anxious to meet it. I put every ounce of strength I had into the project, making a seventy pound pull dogwood bow. Max made a thirty pound pull bow. I wondered why at the time.

My earlier days with the slingshot came to mind, and I thought: Will I be as accurate with a bow and arrow as I used to be with my slingshot? I often went out in back of the house and practiced with the slingshot, and my precision improved greatly.

When the bows were finished, Max took me to the country for target practice. We stopped by a large shaded area, and I felt like Robin Hood as I placed the bow between my feet and pulled the string back with both hands. The bow-string tore at the skin on my kneecap. The arrow hit an old stump going clear through it.

Max took out his handkerchief and bandaged my knee. "Say, that bow is too heavy for you, Russ. Let's swap," he said as his kind eyes searched mine. "I'll even pay you if you do."

I knew then why he had built the lesser bow. He knew I wouldn't be able to handle the monster I had created for myself but he hadn't wanted to discourage me.

"We'll swap even," I said.

He went to the stump and came back. "Your arrow not only went clean through the stump, it also stuck in the ground. You've built some bow, Russ. Yes sir! Some bow!"

I was proud. Max always treated me as an equal. He never once looked down on me. We often hunted together after that and he became my best friend.

The winter of my seventeenth year arrived. It was Sunday, December 7, 1941. I was reading an article in a magazine about the new fad, chess games by mail. Buddy, my parakeet, was perched on my shoulder. The radio was on and all of a sudden the President's voice came over the air and announced that the Japanese had bombed Pearl Harbor and we were at war.

Mom and Dad cried, and I knew they weren't only crying because Bill and Buzz would be involved; they were also crying

THE ROAD BACK

for our country. It was a sad day for all of us, and I'm sure the whole country wept, each individual with his own fears.

Buzz joined the Seabees. He wrote to us as often as he could. Some of his letters were sad and some happy. One day he wrote that he had become champion boxer in his outfit. I didn't doubt this for a minute, the way he used to fight and stick up for me.

Bill and his wife were living in Moline, Illinois, at the time. He had always loved flying, and we supposed he would soon join the Air Force.

After a year of radio news, hearing of some victories and many defeats as the Germans advanced hot and heavy across Europe, the Japanese front also a great threat, I decided to join in the country-wide chess matches by mail I had been reading about. Not too many people in Stanton played chess. It was a small town and checkers prevailed.

I persuaded Dad to bring home a stack of postcards and began the matches, anxiously waiting for my opponents' replies. The postcard chess quotations came rolling in from all over the country

One day there was a knock at the door and Mom answered. The postmaster stood there with two men.

"You have a son named Russell, do you not?" I heard one of them say.

"Why yes," Mom answered.

"We're investigating something which has been called to our attention." I heard the other man say.

Mom asked the two men in. They showed her their identification cards.

The postmaster also stepped inside and stared at me. He had never seen me, and his face wore a puzzled look.

The two investigators approached me. The tall one said, "You have been sending coded messages by postcard all over the country, I hear. What can you tell me about this?"

It was obvious the postmaster did not play chess, and Mom looked at me, a mischievous gleam in her eye. She would enjoy seeing his expression when he learned about the postcards. Many German and Japanese citizens were under suspicion at that time, and being of German descent, Mom resented the accusation.

I had a special chair which Dad had built for me at the time. It had rollers on it and swiveled. I swung the chair around like an executive, then pulled myself along by grasping other pieces of furniture and went to my bedroom, returning with many postcards. I smiled. "These are chess quotations," I said, taking pleasure in their open mouth expressions.

The tall agent took the stack of cards and looked at them. His face became very red and he handed the cards to his associate. Suddenly a roar of laughter rang like freedom bells on a clear cold day as the two investigators admitted the humor of the whole affair.

The poor postmaster stood stroke-like in front of Mom and me, unable to even offer an apology. The mighty keeper of correspondence must be given credit for being on his toes though, but I doubt he ever lived it down after the townfolk got wind of it, because Dad naturally took advantage of the situation. He was determined to avenge the wrong heaped upon his fine upstanding German-American family. This was one time in his life he wasn't so forgiving.

Summer came, and after three months of pleasure with Max Patch—hunting, fishing, building shelves, and making jewelry—the recreation hall closed and we moved to Davenport, Iowa, located on the Mississippi River. Dad lost the election that year and was out of a job. Bill came from Moline, Illinois, to help us move.

The day before we were to leave Bill came running into the house. "Pete's had an accident on his bicycle. He's at the doctor's office—broke his leg!"

"So what's new?" Mom said, as she went on with her packing.

Bill was always teasing, but this time I could tell by the look on his face he wasn't.

"No, Mom," he shouted. "It's true!"

Mom turned around and looked at me, then at Bill. Soon she was out the door with Bill at her heels.

The next day I was stuffed into the car along with poor Pete. Mom, Dad, and Snooky were in the front seat. I was in the back with Pete and his cumbersome cast, holding the birdcage, and little Buddy screeched all the way to Davenport. I guess he didn't want to move either. Bill drove ahead of us, his car loaded with household goods.

As the car bounced along I wondered what Davenport would be like.

"Good job opportunities," Dad said. "I'll surely find work there. Toots and Bill said there are plenty of jobs. After all, that area is a big farm implement center."

After the hot, dusty trip to Davenport and several days of searching, we settled into a small house at the bottom of a park.

It was at this time I faced other problems and decisions, later finding myself enrolled at the Illinois Research Hospital in Chicago.

9 Time of Sadness and Discovery: School for the Handicapped

The move to Davenport was successful, and we began to see better times for awhile. Dad found work in a large farm implement company. It was 1942, and I was eighteen years old.

That fall Pete needed a home tutor for awhile because of his broken leg. She came and decided I should study along with Pete; but little Buddy wouldn't stand for it. He took a dislike to her even though I liked her. We had to put him in his cage each day until she left.

In November I turned nineteen and was only at the level of a fifth grader in academic work, but I was determined to learn. I continued with my home studies, Mom had taught school earlier in her life and now that the rest of her children were away at school, in service, or married, she had time to help me.

Little Buddy would perch on my shoulder as I studied, flying down to pick up pencils and other things I dropped, promptly returning them to me. When I wasn't studying, I taught him other tricks.

One day as he perched on the faucet he slipped and fell into the dishwater. I screamed and Mom came into the kitchen just in time to save him. He was covered with suds. When he dried out enough, he flew to my shoulder, shaking and grateful to be back on his familiar perch. This near-drowning was only a prelude to the real tragedy.

A few weeks later his curiosity and blithe spirit made him venture over to the mousetrap Mom had set. I looked over and was helpless. I couldn't reach him fast enough. He poked his little head into the trap and the trap snapped. I hated my inadequacy, remembering the time the cottonwood tree was struck by lightning. I had been able to escape the tree falling on me and had felt proud that day. But now I judged my theory of being slow but sure to be false. I wasn't able to save my little pet I loved so much. I hated myself.

Mom heard my cries and rushed into the kitchen. I pointed to the trap.

She rushed over and freed Buddy. He flapped his wings several times. Then he rose up from the floor and struggled to find his way to my shoulder once again. After several tries he perched on my shoulder. I saw his head droop and he fell over.

Mom picked him up. "Oh, Russ, he's dead. I'm sorry, so sorry," she cried.

Buddy's death was very difficult to face, and I slumped back into the mire of self-pity.

Soon after this we received word that Buzz was injured—a leg wound.

"Will he be crippled, too?" I wondered with horror. I prayed for his recovery; his leg healed, and he was sent back to his outfit. I thanked the Lord and continued praying for his safety.

Not long after these two sad affairs we received word from Decatur, Nebraska. Grandfather Sears had passed away.

As Mom put down the receiver she leaned on the table, her shoulders slumped, her fingers clutching the phone.

"What's wrong, Mom?" I said.

She turned and faced me. "Your grandfather died—heart attack."

"No! No! No! No! He can't! He couldn't!" I sobbed. It was as if a part of me had died, too.

Mom came over and buried her face in my hair. "Russ, shhh, Russ."

She took her apron and wiped her face. "I'll call your father right away. Come on. You lie down now. There's much to be done."

She helped me into my bed and kissed me on the cheek, her tears mingling with mine.

After a while I couldn't cry anymore. How long I lay in my bed staring at the ceiling I cannot remember. Then little rivulets of tears spilled down over my face, cascading onto my throat as I again choked and fought my sorrow. Life would never be quite the same without my grandfather. He was the one who had insisted I use many tools to make my hands strong. He was the one who had insisted I leave the hospital at Lincoln.

"Why him?" I angrily asked the Lord. "He was a strong man— a useful man. Why not me? Why not me?"

After that I slumped deeper into my dank self-pity. I felt my grandfather's death so greatly I couldn't swallow food for days.

It took me several years to reason why God had not taken me instead of my grandfather. At this time I became twice blessed when my grandfather again helped me to live.

Bill came home on leave. He was in the Air Force. After my grandfather's funeral Bill asked us to move into his house in Moline, Illinois. There was more room, and he asked that Mom care for his daughter while he and his wife were at his air base.

Mom agreed, and we packed up and moved across the Mississippi River into Moline.

After Snooky and Pete were installed at the school, Mom learned of a school for the handicapped located in Rock Island, the town bordering Moline. Arrangements were made for me to attend.

A big black Cadillac picked me up at the house. The driver of the hearse-like limousine was very friendly, and I didn't feel the fear I usually felt when attending a school. I knew there would be others like me, and I looked forward to meeting them.

We collected the other students along the way. "Where are

the boys?" I thought, as the driver helped each girl into the car.

Mary Jane had spastic paralysis. She was beautiful, though, having long dark shiny hair. Her type of spastic paralysis was similar to palsy, and she shook most of the time. She talked very well, though, and was sophisticated.

Shirley had a heart ailment, and one of the other girls suffered from rheumatic fever and also had a heart ailment. Another girl had a brittle bone disease, another a deformity of her hands and legs. A little eight-year-old had the problem of one leg being shorter than the other.

Later others enrolled in the school, including a boy named Teddy. He was ten years younger than I, and he was also saddled with spastic paralysis. I could mirror my own looks through him, and I pitied him. I even dared to interrupt the teacher one day, telling her my grandfather had insisted I use all sorts of tools so my hands wouldn't wither. She took away Teddy's blocks and handed him several tools instead. I helped him and was happy to see him progress as I had done. Teddy had helped me pull myself up from the mire of self-pity I had slipped into.

One hot day I decided to give my schoolmates a treat, and perhaps if I'd known what was to follow I wouldn't have.

More students than usual were placed inside the bus that day when they learned I was going to buy ice cream cones for everyone.

Mary Jane ended up on my lap due to the crowded bus. She squealed with delight over the thought of an ice cream treat as the driver of the bus pulled up to the ice cream store. Mary Jane put her arms around me and hugged me. The close contact triggered a feeling I had only experienced privately, and I tried to control my emotions as best I could. That was the first time any female other than the ones in my family had shown me affection, and I felt like a man. I also became very uncomfortable and embarrassed.

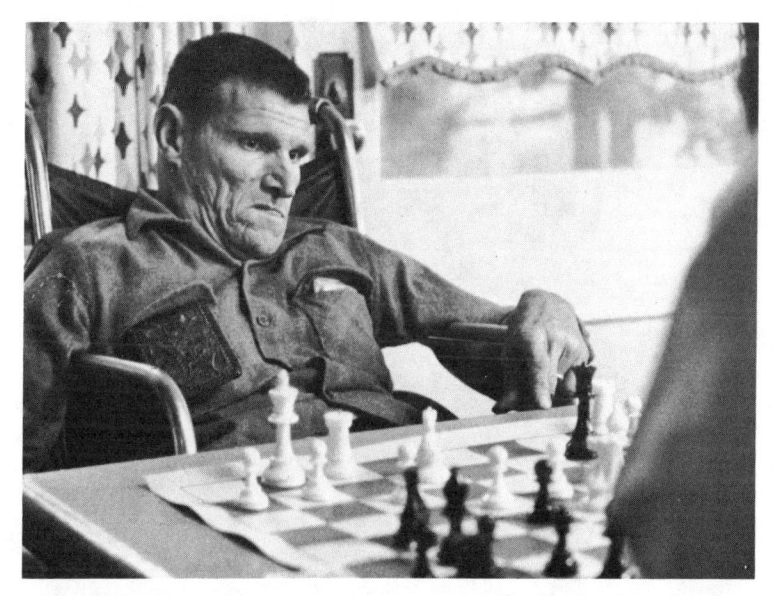

(Top) "Maybe that wasn't such a good move after all," Russell Schultze concedes (*Dispatch* Photo). (Bottom) Kathy and Russell with Willetta J. Balla

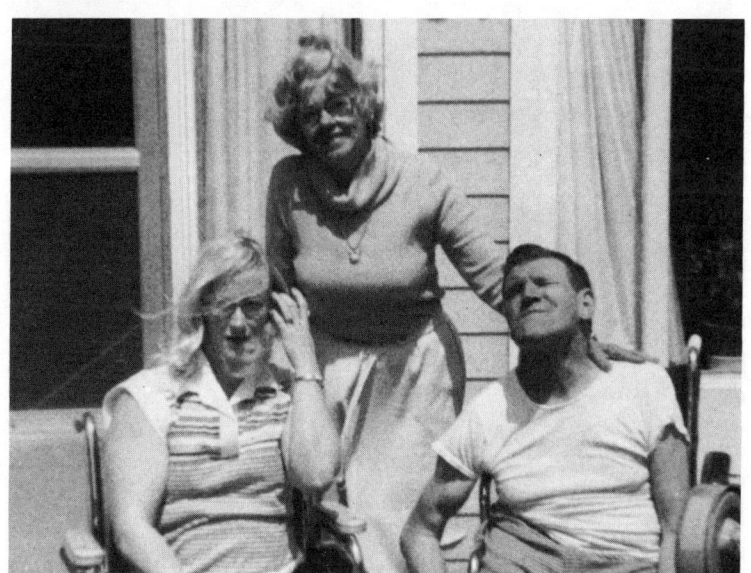

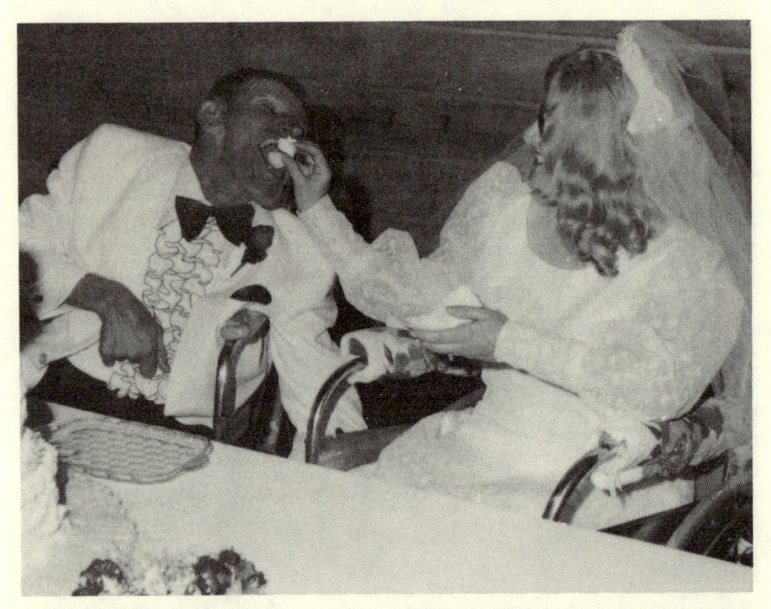

(Top) The traditional "feeding" of the wedding cake (Bottom) Russ in his younger days

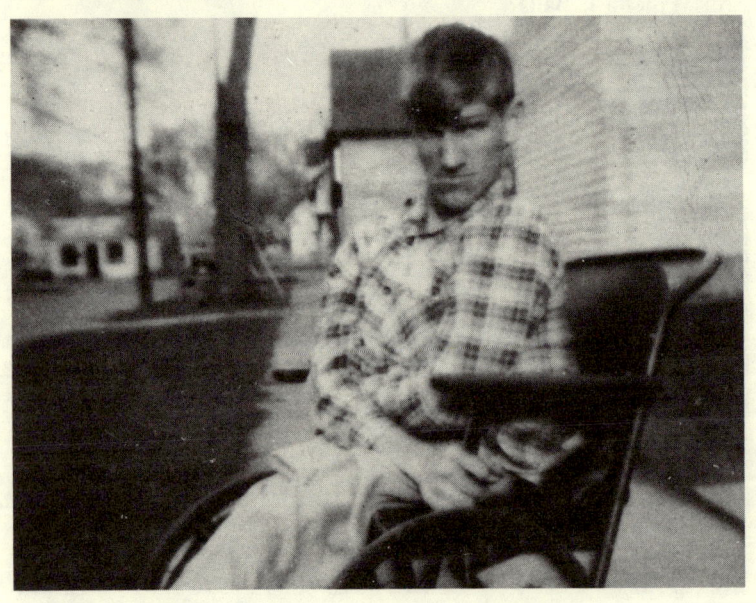

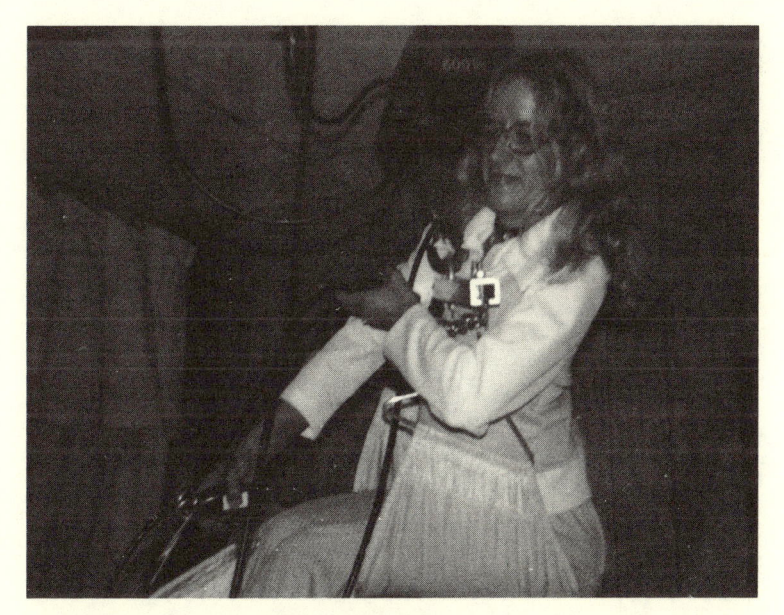

(Top) "Herky," the electric hoist over the Schultzes' bed (Bottom) "Betsy # 7," an electric car built by Russ

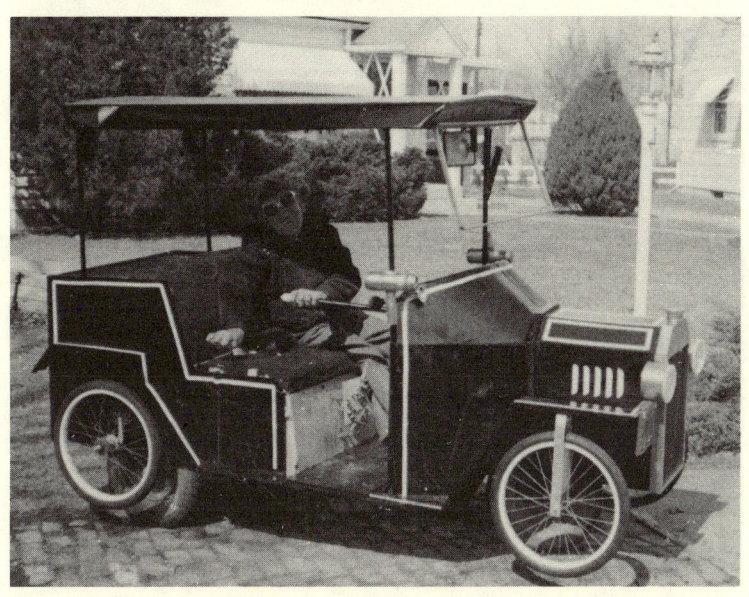

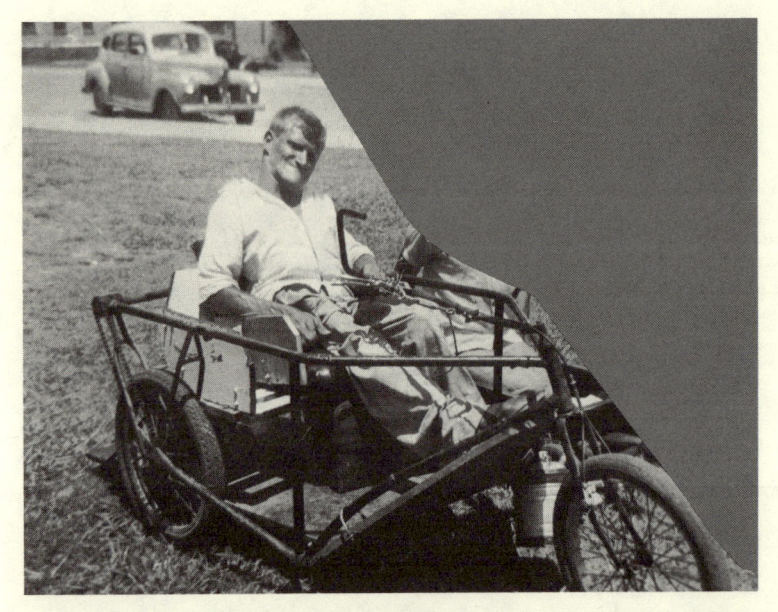

(Top) "Betsy # 1," the heroine of Russ' Arkansas mountain adventure (Bottom) "That's a good one!"

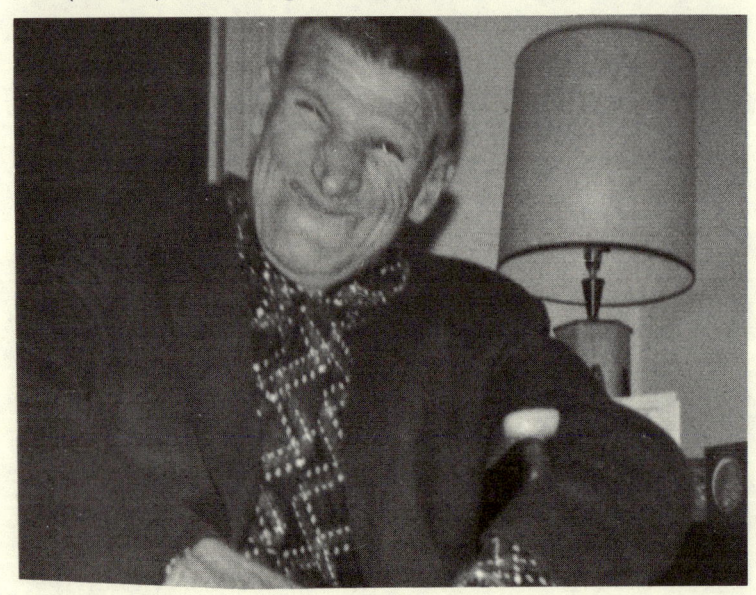

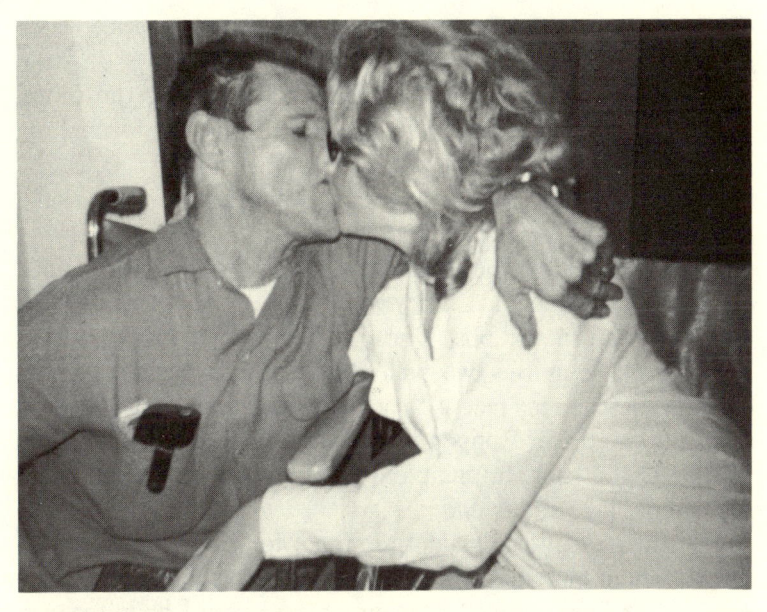

(Top) Russell and Kathy "seal it with a kiss." (Bottom) At work on "Betsy # 11"

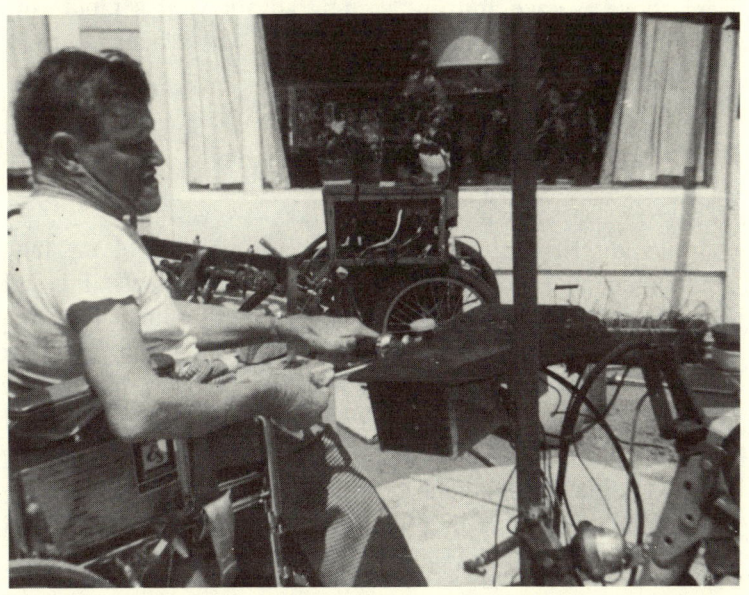

The driver returned with two large trays holding the cones, and I'm sure my ice cream held the record that day for melting the fastest.

That night as I lay in my bed I wondered what it would feel like to hold a girl in my arms.

After that day at the ice cream store my popularity seemed to grow. Mary Jane and Shirley would struggle to see who would sit on my lap in the bus. One day I ended up in the middle of a big battle as the two pulled each other's hair and in the process scratched my face as they fought to see who would occupy my lap. The driver stopped the car and placed Mary Jane and Shirley at the back, bringing one of the younger girls up front. My simple love affairs ended.

I learned many things at the school for the handicapped. I learned about human relationships, applied psychology, and adaptation. I had experienced a feeling of belonging I hadn't experienced before, and I had more confidence in myself. My grades were above average and my learning advanced at a rapid rate. However, at this time my desire to be a whole man returned. I wanted to walk; I wanted to be normal.

One day, soon after my twentieth birthday, the teacher came up to me.

"Russell, this is your special day. The class is at your disposal. Whatever you want to do this afternoon we will do."

I thought this extra fine privilege was because of my high grades, feeling I was being rewarded for my efforts. I didn't know at the time my papers had come from the Illinois Research Hospital in Chicago. I had applied there, hoping if they took me they might be able to help me walk. I felt I must make one last effort to do so and had heard of the free treatment there along with aid in studying. I could finish my schooling there. I knew I would be a guinea pig and face many tests, but I didn't care. I wanted to walk. I wanted to work and get married like everyone else.

After an afternoon of listening to several records I had chosen I requested a very special one. The teacher played *I Love You, Truly*. I had requested it for the girls who had made me feel important—had made me feel like a man. They were all quite a bit younger than I, but they were my first girlfriends, and I loved them dearly.

Then the teacher made the announcement: "This is Russell's last day here at the school. He has been accepted at the Illinois Research Hospital in Chicago. He will be able to graduate from the eighth grade there."

That night as I lay in bed I prayed, "Lord, if it is your will that I walk, please let me. Let my legs move and carry me. Lift this burden from my family. Let me be a whole man!"

10 Hopes and Dreams: My First True Love

In December of my twentieth year, 1944, snow fell softly down over tall buildings and the lights from many cars glistened through the white mist.

The car stopped in front of the research hospital in Chicago. Mom got out and went inside to pave the way for my arrival.

"Russ," Dad said, "are you sure this is what you want?"

Was he thinking of the hospital at Lincoln and the suffering I experienced there as a boy?

"This is what I want, Dad," I answered, as I sat watching the activity around the large hospital entrance. Many patients were leaving to spend the Christmas holiday with their families. I was entering and would not be home for Christmas. I had missed three others, the years I spent at the hospital in Lincoln, but I didn't seem to care. I wanted to walk.

"All right," Dad said, as his gloved fingers fumbled with the steering wheel, "but why couldn't they wait until after Christmas? Besides, I've always provided for you. I don't like this idea of charity—something for nothing."

I leaned forward and patted his shoulder. "Don't worry about it. I'll be fine. The hospital has the vacancy now. I'm twenty years old. Even if I haven't grown very tall, and even if I don't have to shave yet, my mind is grown-up. I want this last chance. I want to walk!"

"I understand," he said angrily. He sighed. "We're here now, and we'll just have to make the best of it. I still don't like the idea of your coming here for nothing though. We have always paid our way! I don't like this idea of a free hospital!"

Mom came through the hospital door with an orderly. The

orderly pushed the chair down the ramp.

I saw he was black. I had never spoken to a black person. He opened the car door and smiled at me. "I'm Jim," he said. "Let's get you inside and get you settled."

"H-e-l-l-o," I stammered.

After he and Dad had pulled me from the car and I was seated in the wheelchair, he spun the chair around, Mom and Dad anxiously following along behind us.

After what seemed like hours, answering questions as the nurse took the necessary information and Dad pacing up and down the hall, Jim came back to take me to my ward.

Dad looked at the nurse. "If you need any money for him I'll pay. I have money to pay!" Mom blushed, then leaned down and kissed me, turned, and did not look my way again.

Dad extended his hand. I took it, and with my own hand, as steady as I could command, squeezed hard. He coughed and sputtered, then followed Mom out of the hospital.

Jim, the orderly, wheeled me into the large lobby. It was filled with happy, babbling people, and a beautiful Christmas tree stood in the center trimmed in red, green, and silver. It was like a beacon offering me hope.

Then a young man hobbled up to it and screamed: "What good is Christmas? I hate it—I hate it all!" He began ripping ornaments off the tree. Pieces of red and green along with strips of tinsel spread out over the floor, his cries of despair hiding the breaking noise.

Two orderlies rushed up to him and pulled him away from the tree. I closed my eyes as we passed by, too sorrowful to watch as they carried him out of the lobby.

This was not a good beginning for me, and all of a sudden I wanted out. I wanted to go home. I felt ashamed. So soon? So soon had I lost my faith again? I felt the motion of my wheelchair, my eyes still closed. Then I felt movement upward.

The elevator suddenly came to a jolting stop. The doors

opened, and another Christmas tree stood tall and proud, its lights seeming to beckon me into my new surroundings.

I straightened up, forced my shoulders back, and looked around. Men in wheelchairs and on crutches were grouped around the tree laughing and joking, and my faith returned along with my spirits.

I didn't mind the skimpy meals the following week. Everything was too new for my appetite anyway. I received brain wave tests, X rays, and a complete checkup, along with many other tests, and I thought, "Well, you asked to be a guinea pig so don't complain."

I enjoyed my studies and also enjoyed the occupational therapy room where I was free to make jewelry and leather goods. I also enjoyed the recreation room on my floor, playing checkers and chess with the other patients. I was kept so busy after the tests that I didn't get homesick.

There was a man in my ward named Joe. He was a real challenge at the checkerboard. We played many games together, and I was delighted whenever I won, but then Joe would be grouchy for hours. He had broken his leg and it never mended right. He was recovering from having it broken and set again. He didn't have the patience I did, but then he wasn't used to his condition.

There was a nurse on the floor named Updike. We got along well together, but she and Joe did not. He was very demanding and didn't get along too well with anyone.

One of the interns watched me play chess one day in the recreation room. I lost the match. The next afternoon when things were slow the intern came into the ward. I was in my bed resting.

He came to my bed. "How would you like to play a game of chess?" he said. "You should keep your hands as busy as you can. I hear you're very good at making jewelry up in therapy. They also tell me you are excellent at making leather purses and wallets—a real whizbang with the featherstitch."

"I'd like a game of chess," I answered. "Where do you want to play, in the therapy room or in the recreation room?"

He helped me into my wheelchair and soon I was inside a large bathroom. He locked the door, took a chessboard from behind the tub and placed it on my lap. Then taking a box from behind the lavatory he opened it and placed the chessmen for me. "I'll play you a dollar a game," he said.

I knew by this time I was being set up, and I had some money Dad left with me.

I won the first game and he seemed quite disturbed.

"Double or nothing on the next game?" he asked anxiously.

"Double or nothing it will be," I answered. I won again.

He couldn't understand how I became so accurate after watching me bungle the game the day before. He didn't know that I had had a headache.

It was getting late. He scooped the chessmen off the board and threw them into the box, folded the board, and hid our secret once again. "We'll continue tonight if you want to, Schultze. How about it? Double or nothing?"

This went on for two nights. I ended up with a hundred dollars, and he was nervous and red in the face. I felt guilty. He was an intern and needed his money. It had been so easy for me. I handed the money back to him. "Don't ever gamble at chess; there's enough gamble in the game itself."

He took the money and left. I never saw him on our floor again. I was angry with myself when I realized I had given him my original dollar. He had beaten me out of a dollar. I learned that sometimes nobody wins.

After a couple of weeks of tests and getting acquainted with the patients in my ward I seemed to settle down into a regular routine. Jim, the orderly, and I were good friends by now.

Late one afternoon as Jim was bringing me back from occupational therapy he asked, "Do you like your ward? Sure are plenty of pretty nurses for you to look at. How many conquests have you made?"

I was somewhat taken back by his bold statement, but at that moment a pretty blond nurse approached us.

"Hello," she said with a flashy white smile. "I'm a student nurse. My name is Mary Ellen Eike, and I've been assigned to you, I believe. Russell Schultze is it?" She looked at the chart.

"Thanks, Jim," she said. "Has a Mr. Jason Smithfield arrived yet?"

"No," he answered, "Smithfield won't be coming in until Monday."

"Well, take Mr. Schultze to his ward," she replied as she smiled down at me, placing her hand on my shoulder. "I'll come in and check you later, Mr. Schultze."

She turned and I watched her walk away, my heart seeming to leap right into my throat. She was a vision with silky blond hair, short in stature, blue eyes, dimples, and a very slim but well-proportioned body. She had called me Mr. Schultze. I didn't even remember being pushed into the ward with its many beds.

After I was settled, Mary Ellen entered the ward. My heart jumped again.

She smiled, took her blood pressure kit and opened it, placed the wide band around my arm, and began pumping. I felt a pounding in my chest and I'm sure my breathing was rapid.

"You're a little excited tonight, but a good night's sleep will take care of that," she said as she placed a thermometer in my mouth and took my hand, pressing her slender fingers into my wrist.

"I'll get an order from the doctor and see that you get something to calm you down."

Little did she know at the time that the increased blood pressure and the rapid pulse was because of her. Then she left me, returning later with a pill. I obediently took it and soon I was drowsy. I closed my eyes to the checker players and everything else around me and drifted into a valley of pleasant dreams.

The following day I was subjected to more tests and one of them disturbed me greatly. They tried to hypnotize me but the test failed. I resented someone trying to capture my mind. I had struggled too hard to get it back and didn't want anyone fooling with it. It was working good and I wanted to keep it that way.

"Why did they try to hypnotize me?" I said to Mary Ellen that afternoon as she was taking my pulse.

"It was to see if your illness might possibly be psychosomatic."

"What in heaven's name is that?" I almost shouted. "It sounds terrible."

She laughed. "It means physical ailments due to emotional causes."

"Do they think I'm crazy?" I scolded, disgusted and alarmed. "I was born this way! Don't they know what spastic paralysis is? Didn't they get my papers from the hospital at Lincoln, Nebraska?"

"You ask too many questions, Mr. Schultze," she answered. "And I see I have answered too many. Of course they have your records. And they most certainly know what spastic paralysis is!"

She was angry with me. I hadn't intended to make her angry. "What is your nationality?" I asked, hoping to smooth out her anger some by changing the subject.

"I'm Dutch!" She whipped open her blood pressure kit.

"I'm German all the way through," I teased, "but don't hold it against me. I can't help it if the Germans took over Holland."

Her lips spread into a mischievous smile and two dimples appeared. "Beware if you are ever in need of a shot."

I laughed. "Mary Ellen Eike," I said smugly, as she pumped up the band on my arm.

"Russell Schultze," she answered. "If you ever do need a shot, I promise I'll place the needle carefully. Friends?"

"Friends," I returned.

She packed up her kit and left the room. She had fire! She was just like Mom. She had spirit and was stubborn.

As the months passed we chided each other often, enjoying our parries and thrusts with the language.

I had the only radio in the ward, and I became the hub of much of the activity. We listened to programs along with many interruptions as the newscasters kept the country informed on the latest war news. It was March 1945, and we had the Germans on the run, expecting to hear of their surrender at any time.

One day a doctor came in and told me I was to undergo surgery and my heart sank. Could I take it?

"You'll be in a cast for awhile," he said. "We're going to cut the cords at the back of your knees and try to straighten your legs. There will also be some surgery on your adductor muscles which we hope will keep your knees from rubbing together. Get lots of rest. We've scheduled your surgery two days from today."

His mentioning a cast brought back memories of Lincoln, Nebraska, and the terror and pain I had experienced there. The surgery had to be postponed. My mustard seed eluded me once again, and my temperature climbed along with my blood pressure.

Mary Ellen and the other nurses including Updike would come to me, sometimes in a group and sometimes one by one. They encouraged me, saying: "You'll be fine, Russ. We won't let anything happen to you. Besides, if we did, we would get fired." They would tease and try to lift my spirits.

But as I lay thinking about the surgery I also prayed for courage, and I thought about the others with my type spastic paralysis. Many might walk if my surgery were a success. I searched again for my mustard seed, found it, and it helped me pass over my anxiety.

The surgery was performed, and for the first week I slept

most of the time, free most of the time from pain, later realizing I was on hard drugs.

I demanded to see Nurse Gunther.

"No more drugs!" I shouted. "Didn't my papers say I was a drug addict once? No more drugs!"

She left the room and returned with the doctor. He looked at me sympathetically. "You need these for pain," he said, giving my shoulder a reassuring pat. "Don't worry, we'll make sure you don't acquire the habit again."

"I'll take nothing!" I shouted as a sharp pain shot through me. "I don't want anything. I'll be all right!"

I suffered for several days without anything for the pain. I didn't scream, because I didn't want to disturb the other patients. My eyes, though, and the strained look on my face, along with my almost constant groaning, became too much for Mary Ellen.

"Russ," she begged, "please let the doctors give you something!"

I gave in, and she returned with Miss Gunther.

"Here," Miss Gunther said as she handed me a small cup along with a glass of orange juice. "Drink this fast and wash it down with the juice."

I drank the foul liquid and it burned all the way down as I shivered and shook. But sooner than I expected I fell into a deep sleep, later learning I had taken a drug called paraldehyde. It was not supposed to be habit-forming.

Somehow the drug depressed me. When I was awake, I worried about being able to walk. My faith seemed to slip from me. Something told me I would never walk. I refused to eat and grew weaker each day. I didn't seem to care about anything anymore.

When Mary Ellen was off duty, she would sit by my bed. She was a regular nurse by this time and spent many extra hours taking care of me, holding my hand with tears in her eyes. But I couldn't climb up out of my depression, and I prayed to die.

But just before dawn one morning as Mary Ellen sat with me she patted my hand and said, "Russ, I'm going to go work on the charts now. You try to sleep. I'll be back as soon as I can." She left, and the ward was quiet except for the heavy breathing of the other patients.

I lay thinking about death, surrendering myself to the other side of life I believed in.

Suddenly a booming voice seemed to echo around the ward.

"Why are you giving up? I have given you life. It is my privilege to take it. Not yours!"

Tears spilled from my eyes. "You have not made me perfect! You have not made me walk!"

Then the voice sternly said:

"You will be provided with transportation that you create yourself!"

Then I heard another voice. It was the voice of my grandfather, and I heard him say:

"Come with me, Russ."

I felt myself lifted up, and I looked down onto my misty body, feeling myself floating off and away. I could see the earth below me. Do these things happen? They did to me.

Then grandfather said: "This is what will happen."

I felt his hand touch mine as we watched the earth stretch out like a large long watermelon as it spun. The earth began to separate, and it seemed many people were clambering to get back where they belonged. Then the earth completly separated, and one part became engulfed in a fleecy white cloud.

My voice sounded far off as I asked: "When is this to happen?"

"I cannot say. You should not ask," my grandfather said.

I saw the earth come together again, and soon I was drifting back, my grandfather still holding my hand. We seemed to zero in on the hospital, going right through walls, and I drifted into the ward and saw my body in the bed beneath me.

Then grandfather said: "It is not your time, Russ. You must

store up more knowledge on this earth learning about your Master."

It felt as if I were rubbing against sandpaper as I slipped back into my body. I lay in a cold sweat, knowing I hadn't dreamed that experience.

Mary Ellen returned soon after, and I told her about the experience.

She threw herself over me and cried. "See, Russ? You have to get well!"

After that early dawn experience I began to recover in spite of myself, struggling with the pain and discomfort, and my appetite returned. I grew stronger each day.

The German surrender came, and I was grateful I hadn't been allowed to surrender myself.

June came, and whenever Mary Ellen could find the time she would take me to the roof of the hospital, bed and all.

One warm sunny day she came up to me as I was struggling over a checker game with Joe.

"Come on, Russell Schultze, I'm taking you up onto the roof. You're as pale as a ghost. Be ready in ten minutes; I'll collect you then." She left and naturally I lost the checker game.

I took my mirror from my nightstand and looked into it. I was discouraged. There wasn't a whisker on my face yet, and I was going to be twenty-one in November. It was the middle of June, and it looked as though I would never grow hair on my face.

As I studied the mirror I saw a pale man with a determined chin, blue eyes, and sandy hair. I decided then and there I wasn't handsome but that I wasn't ugly either. This was the kindest thought I ever had about myself at that time. I liked me. I liked Mary Ellen, and she liked me. This was all that seemed to matter.

The hospital roof was empty as we entered it except for a few men at one end and a girl with a nurse reading her some mail. The girl had a patch over one eye. Other than that we were alone.

Mary Ellen tucked my blanket around my legs and sat in a chair beside the bed. She opened a book of poetry.

"Oh, no," I sighed. "You're not going to read that silly stuff to me are you?"

"Indeed I am. Your teacher told me you must have this if you want to be a well-rounded student. You want to graduate don't you?"

"Oh, well," I said, "I guess I can stand it if you read it to me."

"Are you familiar with Scott?" she said as she opened the white hand-tooled book cover with a pale pink rose also etched on it.

"Who's he?" I asked, giving her a devil-may-care smile.

"Now stop that!" she scolded, as she turned several pages. "I'm going to read parts of Scott's *Lady of the Lake*. It's my favorite."

She began, and to this day I love poetry. Her voice was very soft, inviting me into a new mood, a mood of dreaminess, far more pleasant than any drug as she read:

> A while the maid the stranger eyed,
> And, reassured, at length replied,
> That Highland halls were open still
> To wilder'd wanderers of the hill.
> Nor think you unexpected come
> To yon lone isle, our desert home;
> Before the heath had lost the dew,
> This morn, a couch was pull'd for you;
> On yonder mountain's purple head
> Have ptarmigan and heath-cock bled,
> And our broad nets have swept the mere
> To furnish forth your evening cheer.

I reached over, hand calm, and took her's in mine. "That's really beautiful, Mary Ellen. I honestly liked it."

She smiled. "Now, I'll give you another dose."

I watched as her soft delicate hands turned a few pages.

> The mistress of the mansion came,
> Mature of age, a graceful dame;
> Whose easy step and stately port
> Had well become a princely court,
> To whom, though more than kindred knew,
> Young Ellen gave a mother's due.
> Meet welcome to her guest she made,
> And every courteous rite was paid,
> That hospitality could claim,
> Though all unask'd his birth and name.

She looked up and saw my tears. "Why Russell, you do love poetry as I do."

"I love you!" I had spit out the words so quickly I couldn't believe it was me.

She laid the book on the bed, stood, and put her arms around me, kissing me on both cheeks as if to kiss my tears away.

That afternoon I was swept into a peaceful valley as I lay holding her hand, the sun and her nearness flooding me with warmth.

Then it was time to leave, and I listened to her soft steps as she pushed me into the elevator, feeling the sun leave my back and shoulders, but the warmth I felt inside remained.

Two weeks later we were truly in love. I was happy, happier than I had ever been. I decided to make her a fine leather purse with a wallet to match.

When I wasn't in occupational therapy, my fingers weaving the leather strips in and out at the edges of the purse, I continued with my chess and checker games in the ward or listened to the radio. We were in real trouble with the Japanese by then, and it seemed the war would never end.

One day, as I was playing a game of checkers with Joe, both of us straining over the few checkers left on the board, Joe made a move, then growled: "Stay away from Mary Ellen! She's mine, and I heard about the purse you're making for her."

I thought he was trying to distract me.

"I'm dead serious," he said. "Keep your cotton pickin' hands off Mary Ellen!"

All of a sudden I felt like Caesar our bull. I saw red, and I wanted to wrap his wheelchair around his neck.

"What's your pleasure?" I snorted. "Slingshots at twenty paces? Stilettos with one hand tied behind us, or do you want to settle this over the checkerboard?"

"OK," he returned. "Checkers! Winner take all!"

Before I knew it he pulled out a coin. "Heads or tails?"

"Heads!" I snapped in anger. "What have I done?" I thought as the coin landed on the wrong side, leaving me the red checkers and Joe the privilege to choose his own opening.

Mary Ellen came into the ward. "Come on everybody. It's lights out."

She walked up to us. "Feeling pretty good tonight, aren't you, Russ? Your face has some real color to it. I'm glad to see the good food and good care helped put it there."

Joe grabbed her arm. "Hi, sweetie." He pressed his fingers into her soft flesh, and I wanted to kill him.

"Take your hands off her!" I shouted.

"All right!" Mary Ellen scolded. "You two have been together too long today. Russ, you get those hands of yours moving and wheel yourself over there to that bed right now! Come on, Joe, here's your night pill. Take it and hop up on the bed or I'll call an orderly!"

Joe gave me a sarcastic grin. "Russ and I have a big day tomorrow. Yes sir, a big day. We've got a big tournament on—

one heck of a big tournament, sweets, and it's winner take all!"

I whirled around in my wheelchair and went to my bed thinking how ridiculous I had been by losing my temper and getting myself into a situation that might prevent me from being close to Mary Ellen. I took all games seriously by then, and I would have to stay away from her if I lost.

Mary Ellen helped me into bed. "What's wrong, Russ? You're all upset. Don't let Joe get to you. You know how he is. Do you want a sleeping pill?"

"No. I won't need it. I'll be fine," I lied as she tucked me beneath the covers. I slept poorly.

The next day the two pale knights dressed in their hospital battle fatigues took off across the checkerboard, minds sharp, visions clear, fleshy lances extended as they attacked the red and black armies. We decided two out of three wins would determine the victor.

Some of the other patients in the ward had heard us quarreling over Mary Ellen, and before we finished the first game we were surrounded by onlookers. Most of the patients in the ward were on hand to see who would win the fair Ellen.

Three days passed. The men crowded around us and we were both on edge. On the fourth day we decided that after lunch we would slip from the ward and finish our battle beside the fountain outside the hospital. When the others settled down for a rest, we left the ward separately. This was our last game, and whoever won also won Mary Ellen.

I thought: "How foolish this is. How could two grown men get themselves into such a ridiculous situation?"

"Well move!" Joe shouted, the water from the fountain spouting, then making an annoying trickling sound. A statue of a naked man stood in the center of the fountain, our only onlooker.

My hand shook as I made my next move. It was a stupid one, and Joe skipped over three of my men, then took his cane from the arm of his wheelchair and gleefully banged it on the side of the fountain. "Looks like Mary Ellen won't have to wait for me much longer." He gave me a smug grin.

I heard the babble of voices, looked up, and two interns followed by several of the patients in our ward were approaching. Before we knew it we were again surrounded by spectators. Jim, the orderly, and even Nurse Updike ended up in the audience.

I made my next move and looked for Mary Ellen. She wasn't in the crowd, and I was grateful, hoping she hadn't heard about our silly tournament. When I looked at the board again I was down another checker.

All of a sudden Updike leaned over, the breeze making her hair fall and tickle Joe's neck.

Joe became restless and shook his shoulders saying: "Go get me a cup of coffee, someone."

"I'll have a glass of water," I added.

Updike left to bring us our time-out refreshment.

Mary Ellen returned with her. I was ashamed. I felt like a little boy instead of a man.

There were only a few checkers left on the board. Updike was about to hand Joe his coffee when she tipped the cup forward. The coffee spilled into his lap. He jumped, and Mary Ellen took the glass of water and poured it on top of the coffee stain. Then Joe, quite unnerved, pushed the wrong checker, and I won. He bolted from his chair, the checker board flying into the air, and the statue received a good whack on its bare rump as Joe's cane came down across it. Joe hobbled back up the hospital lawn, spouting fiery words like an erupting volcano.

I looked up at Mary Ellen and she was smiling. It was then I knew she had planned to upset the game. Her eyes twinkled, and Updike shook with laughter.

"Come on, Russ," Mary Ellen said, as she turned my wheelchair around.

"How did you know?" I questioned, as the spectators spread out over the lawn on their way back to the hospital.

She flicked me on the back of my neck with her fingers. "Those men in the ward are worse than a flock of gossiping old women; that's how. Russell Schultze, you're impossible!"

I listened as she clucked all the way back to the hospital like a little bantam hen. I was happy. The knight or whatever I thought of myself then had won his lady fair, and that night young Ellen paid me every courteous rite, the hospitality of her warm lips on mine in the quiet darkness of the ward.

I remembered Mary Jane at the school for the handicapped and how I felt when she sat on my lap in the limousine, remembering the want I experienced then. Now my feelings were stronger. I wanted Mary Ellen, wanted to hold her, wanted to kiss her. Soon she left me and I couldn't sleep. I lay trembling with desire. She had asked me to marry her, telling me she loved me, and wanted to take care of me. I knew I could not marry her. I couldn't let her tie herself down to a cripple; I loved her too much for that. It wouldn't be fair to her.

The day I finished the purse and wallet I tucked the wallet inside the purse and left the therapy room, knowing by then they were to be a parting gift. My studies were finished, and I was to graduate the following day.

I asked Mary Ellen to meet me up on the roof at three o'clock. It was ten minutes to three as the elevator door opened. She was there waiting for me.

"So sad, Russ?" she said, as I looked up into her face.

I handed her the purse. "This is for you, Mary Ellen. It's a parting gift made with love."

She took the purse from my shaking hands. "Oh, Russ, it's beautiful!"

"Look inside," I said, as I fought my sorrow. "There's a wallet to match."

She opened the purse and took out the wallet, her tears making dark marks on the leather. Then she knelt beside me.

"Please Russ, marry me. I love you. Please let me take care of you. I love you so."

The interruption of passersby gave me time to collect my reason.

"I won't let you spend your life taking care of me!" I shouted. "I can't support you, and I love you too much. I can't marry you! I'd hate myself if I did. I won't let you bind yourself to a life of service to me!"

My hands gripped the wheels of my chair and I whirled around, angry, hurt, and sick as I pressed the button at the side of the elevator doors. The doors opened, and I was greatly relieved for the swift deliverance down to my floor, hurriedly seeking the quiet of the washroom.

"It's over," I said as I looked at my face in the mirror. "Russell Schultze, it's over!"

The graduation exercises took place the following day. Mary Ellen didn't show up for the ceremonies and I never saw her again, later regretting I hadn't left myself in her care.

11 The Adjustment: A Search for Happiness

I returned to Moline a stranger in a new neighborhood. Mom and Dad had purchased a house in the uptown district.

On August 14th the Japanese surrendered, and the war was over.

I ignored Mary Ellen's letters, determined she would not tie herself down. It was a very painful experience. I loved her and wanted her, yet I felt she deserved a much better life than I could give her. The letters continued for awhile. Then she stopped writing, and it was easier to get my mind off of her.

The only pleasure I had was when I ventured down to the nearby fire station after I made myself a crude tricycle contraption with a hand crank and a motor. The Lord had told me I must supply my own transportation and I was bound and determined to obey him.

The firemen became good friends of mine, and I enjoyed playing chess and checkers with them. At this time in my life I imagined the only excitement and pleasure I would ever have was the satisfaction I received when I won.

I still yearned for love. I wanted to hold a woman in my arms, loving her the way I knew my brothers loved their wives.

I decided to study electronics. This would take my mind off my problems, too. I knew I had to keep busy. I studied hard and began struggling with amateur inventions. I continued visiting my firemen friends, and their companionship meant everything to me.

Then my Dad bought me an electric shopper car. It was silent, and I got around the Quad Cities with great ease. I heard about the chess tournaments being played at the civic center in Rock

Island, and I drove my electronic car there, finding another release for my pent-up emotions. I was on hand for all the tournaments and became quite well-known there.

My sister Snooky bought me an electric wheelchair one day. I was thrilled with it. There would be no more pushing of wheels in order to get around the house. I thanked the Lord for these two precious gifts of transportation. My shopper car carried me down the streets, and the electric wheelchair also let me get around with ease.

However, one day something went wrong with the electric charger. I struggled trying to fix it but was unsuccessful. I took the charger and went down to the fire station hoping Pete, one of my firemen friends, could help me fix it.

I entered the station and found him polishing the big truck. "Can you help me fix this charger?" I asked.

He lit a cigarette and walked over to me. "Sure will give it a try, Russ," he said, giving me his usual broad grin.

He searched the charger over and removed a pin from it. "You need a new giggling pin, Russ. Try the gas station. I'm sure Bob has one."

I went to the station and asked my friend Bob.

"Sorry, Russ." He smiled. "I'm all out of them. Try the drugstore. Ask Dick. He'll fix you up."

I hurried to the drugstore. My friend Dick went to the back of the store then returned. "Sold the last one yesterday, I guess. Sorry, Russ, but you might find one at the variety store next door."

I was unsuccessful once more. As I came out of the variety store, a man who also frequented the fire station stopped me and said: "Hear you're having trouble with your electric charger." He started to laugh, leaned against the building and slapped his thighs as his laughter increased.

I wanted to crawl into the big crack in the sidewalk, knowing by then it was all a joke. I was angry at first until I too saw

THE ADJUSTMENT

the humor of it all and decided to pay my friend Pete back. Giggling pin? I'd see him not giggling very soon.

Returning to the drugstore, I entered and found Dick.

"Say, can you fix me up fast with four malts? I know what you guys have been up to, and I want to play a trick on Pete. Put a good physic in one of the malts and mark the lid."

He laughed. "I'll fix you up right away, Russ. I'd like to see Pete's face when he discovers what you did to him."

I returned to the fire station, the coldness of the malts reaching through the paper sack and chilling my lap.

Pete and the others were pleased I had taken the joke so well. Pete grabbed the sack from me and distributed the malts. Lids flew. All I could do was accept my fate.

"Oh, well," I thought, "I've got three chances out of four." Several hours later I knew I had lost, and this experience most certainly prompted me into rapid advancement with my electronics studies. I would fix my own electrical failures or die trying!

I put in many hours of study after that and even designed a few small electrical gadgets.

Between my frequent trips to the civic center and the fire station I met a policeman named Frank. He visited the fire station often, and we became good friends. I liked him from the first day we sat and talked. He reminded me of Max Patch, the man at the WPA recreational center in Stanton who had been so kind to me. Frank treated me as an equal, as Max had done.

As our friendship grew he confided in me often, telling me of his worry over the rising delinquency, calling the boys and girls who had gotten themselves into trouble his *kids of the streets*.

One day as we sat over a chess game, the worst game he had ever played, I said: "What's wrong, Frank? You can't even tell the black men from the white. Play with your own men!"

"I'm plenty upset, Russ," he answered. "The growing drug

problem around this area is unbelievable. There are so many pushers getting to my *kids of the streets*, I'll not be surprised if I find out they all take the stuff."

"Let me help, Frank. Let me at least try," I begged.

I told him about my drug experience when I was thirteen.

"Please, Frank, let me help. Send the kids to the civic center in Rock Island. I'll keep them off the streets. I'll teach them chess."

He laughed, then apologized. "Russ, you don't understand. I'm sorry, but I doubt if any of those kids would want to play chess. They would probably laugh. They're tough. They'd think it was a sissy's game."

"Listen, Frank," I continued, "I've played many a chess game with tough guys, and you know it isn't a sissy game."

He placed his hand on my arm. "All right, Russ, I'll see what I can do, but I'll have to talk it over with the probation officer first."

My plea became a reality and some of his boys did come to the center. I began teaching the rascals, and most of them showed a real interest in the game. I also noticed that most of them had keen minds.

By now Mary Ellen was pushed to the back of my mind, and I became wrapped up in my new life.

Then one day I received a letter from the hospital in Chicago. They wanted me back for a checkup. I wondered if Mary Ellen would still be there. What would I say to her? I thought about our times together and became restless. I wanted to see her. Maybe I had been wrong about refusing to marry her.

"Is she happy?" I asked myself. Then I realized I was talking myself into marrying her. I could not support myself or her. Just a quick hello and good-bye was all there could be to it. I would again have to pass up my chance for love.

A few days later I entered the hospital, wanting to see her and nervously planning what I would say.

THE ADJUSTMENT 103

"I'll just have to act as though I'm completely at ease and happy over my circumstances. I'll just tell her I'm very involved in my new life of helping delinquent children and have no time for anything else. That's not too much of a lie," I reasoned.

Nurse Updike spotted me and stopped. "Well, Russ, you look well, very well."

"I'm fine," I returned, as I looked around for Mary Ellen.

Updike placed her hand on my shoulder. "Russ, Mary Ellen isn't here anymore. She joined a group of nurses and went to Africa to do some research . . . she . . ."

"Is she happy?" I asked.

"Russ, I'm sorry," she answered with tears in her eyes. "She joined a leper colony. She died of leprosy. I'm so sorry."

I clutched the arms of my wheelchair, and all I could see was Mary Ellen turning ugly before my eyes, a heavy bell around her neck warning others to stay away as she rotted.

My Lady of the Lake was gone!

I remembered the poem she read to me. Had anybody prepared a couch for her? Had anyone "swept the mere," offering her an evening's cheer?

I returned to Moline a man of stone. As the weeks and months passed, I became more and more despondent. If I had married her, she would be alive and I wouldn't be bearing the terrible guilt I felt. At that time I hated myself. Had I been selfish, caring only about my own feelings—a cripple—unable to support a wife—people whispering, "What does she see in him?" I became so mixed up in my thoughts I was miserable. I had to get away. I had to find answers. I wanted freedom. I wanted to escape from my wheelchair.

"Why me?" I again questioned. "Why was I born a cripple?" Nothing made sense.

That was the summer I went to Mena, Arkansas, to care for Toots' children while she worked.

I returned that fall after my experience in the mountains,

the experience of seeing my grandfather's face through the trees when I sat desolate and alone waiting to be rescued from the terrors of the night. Twice my grandfather's strange appearance had lifted me up, giving me hope, once in those mountains and once at the hospital in Chicago. I felt ashamed. How could I have lost my faith after two such enlightening miracles?

I pushed through my mountain of shame by becoming a searcher for a stronger faith. I visited many churches and studied the Bible. I came to the understanding that no matter what my circumstances were, crippled or strong and perfect of body, I had a place in the world, a cross to bear, and an inborn desire for life after death. God had plans for me, and I knew it!

I became wrapped up in my work with Frank's kids of the streets, teaching them chess and handicrafts at the center in Rock Island. Often they would come to my house and visit.

I had improved greatly in my study of electronics and decided to build myself a special golf car. I didn't play golf, but the car would offer me more speed. Frank was pleased over my helping him with the kids of the streets, and I felt a sturdier vehicle was necessary. Little did I know at the time how necessary it was.

Pete and the other firemen were impressed with my ideas for a design and wanted to help me build the car.

When the design was finished, we sent it along with an order to a large golf-cart firm, feeling we should because they could help us decide on the special parts we needed.

A few weeks later they sent us several hundred dollars worth of parts free, along with a paper to sign. We were so happy with the free parts we signed the design over to them.

When my car was finished, I had the first model of a very fine golf car, and they had the patent. But later I discovered far more wealth than owning a patent on a golf car.

My little car was something, and I named her Betsy, the name I had also given the electric shopper my father had bought

THE ADJUSTMENT

for me. All of my cars were named Betsy after that.

I continued helping Frank with his kids, but the drug traffic increased. Trying to just keep the kids off the streets wasn't enough. I argued with Frank to let me help with the drug problem. He kept refusing because of the danger involved.

The manager of the nearby theater, Buster Brotman, became a good friend of mine. He allowed me to take Frank's kids to the shows free. I gathered kids like moths to a flame after that.

One day a big boy came into the center in Rock Island. He was one of Frank's boys. He was seventeen, six foot one, and weighed about two hundred ten pounds—a real blockbuster.

There was an immediate camaraderie between us. He was strong and I was weak, but he must have admired my ability at the chessboard. He became my most astute pupil.

One day I had his king well-pinned, trying to show him the defensive game of chess. He was quite a bragger and said: "I'm just tired today. Can't think. What a time I had last night. I was hung high. That locoweed and the other goodies were sure something."

"Come on, Jack," I said. "You surely aren't dumb enough to be on that stuff. Make your move."

"So I'm not!" he snapped. "But I know there's plenty to be had. It's all over the school. You can make a buy as easy as the purchase of a pencil."

I looked at his strong, healthy body. Was his bragging a plea for help? Was he tempted but didn't know whether he wanted to join the others who had surrendered themselves into hell? My interest rose as I thought about the two years I spent fighting off the habit I had acquired. I felt sick over the thought of others who were suffering, their bodies drawn up in a fetal position as they shook and screamed for relief. I decided to help stop the drug traffic whether Frank liked it or not. There would be no crystalline armies or split cars running over my kids at the center.

"Come on, Jack," I said. "If you know so much, tell me about it. If you don't take the stuff, do you want your friends to become hooked?"

I told him about my own experience with drugs. "Now do you see why I want to help put an end to this drug traffic? I can do it, too. Come on, Jack, make your move."

He looked down at his pinned king then at me. "I don't know too much about it, but some of us guys could keep our eyes open for you."

I smiled. "You do that, Jack. Come on, make your move, and as long as you offered to help the cause I'll give you a clue. Check out your knights there for a block."

Jack came through for me, and I found myself with several pawns—boys who also wanted to help. I put them into action at the school. They were to watch for any drug traffic and tell me which kids were buying.

I told Frank what I had done, and naturally he was mad.

"You're crazy, Russ! This is a dangerous business. For a filthy buck those pushers will kill! Keep your nose out of it."

"Look, Frank," I pleaded, "you know all about my life. I'm not going to sit here in this wheelchair and allow those people to suck everything good out of your kids of the streets! Please let me do this. I'll do it anyway; you know that."

He yelled: "You stubborn German! I know you will. But at least let me get you some protection. Sometimes I wish I had never met you. You're nothing but a stubborn German!"

"Thanks." I smiled. "I'll be all right. I'm not afraid of those pushers or the man at the top."

He paced up and down the fire station a few times. "Oh, come on! Let's get out of here. I'll get you some help while you play this game, but you better be as good at it as you are at chess or you may end up pinned and checkmated!"

"I'm not worried," I said bravely, already feeling the flesh crawl on my arms and legs. I smiled weakly this time. "Don't

THE ADJUSTMENT

worry about me, Frank. I have a guardian angel on my shoulder, and I'm grateful for the chance to help." The thought of a guardian angel on my shoulder seemed to lessen my anxiety.

He gave me a light punch on my jaw. "You're nuts, Russ, you know that? Watch that guardian angel doesn't get knocked off!"

A couple of days later, as my pawns at the school continued their probe, Frank put his knights at the police station to work, and I became a searching bishop. It wasn't long before Jack and some of his friends at the school told me where to go and witness a buy.

I used my electric shopper car because it was silent. I entered an alley around four o'clock the following morning and turned my lights out. There was an old garage with no doors, and I backed into it. I sat there thinking: "What will you do if a car really does come down this alley and you find your pusher? What next, Russell Schultze? Will you be able to take it? Will you be able to cope with your spastic nerves, or will your body go into a spastic fit? The noise you might make—what about the noise if you jerk all over the place?"

I wanted to leave then and there. I looked out and up at the sky. There was no moon, but the stars shone brightly. "Lord! Give me courage," I prayed.

Suddenly I felt a tickle, then a sting on my arm. "Mosquitoes!" I said in disgust.

They swarmed over my face and arms. Perhaps this was a good thing. I could only think about the miserable insects, shaking and trying to keep up with their constant landings, as I swatted and tried to control my jumping muscles while the tiny pests picked away at my flesh.

Suddenly a car turned into the alley and stopped a few feet from the open garage. There would be no more swatting of mosquitoes. I sat rigid, teeth clenched, and it seemed I felt the prick of a thousand needles as the tiny army finished their meal. I looked down at my white shirt. Would the driver of the car spot it? Stupid! I silently scolded. Why didn't you dress in black?

Then a second car came down the alley, and the lights from it flashed onto the first car. I struggled with my pencil and pad and wrote down the license number. A boy got out of the second car and joined the man in the first one. I witnessed the buy.

Shortly after the two cars drove away two more cars came into the alley. I took down the second pusher's number. I began to wonder just how many pushers there were in our town.

The following day I took the license numbers to Frank, and it wasn't long before we knew who the two pushers were. Frank's knights followed the pushers and found they frequented a tavern not far from the fire station.

I had some trouble with Mom at this time. She worried about my being out at all hours of the night. I didn't want to alarm her and told her I liked to play chess with the firemen at night because it helped them pass many hours of boredom.

"Well," she scolded, "they should keep their doors shut at night. Look at your face and arms. They're covered with bites. It's a terrible year for mosquitoes, and they should know better!"

My witnessing a buy wasn't enough, according to Frank. The authorities would have to also witness one. Frank wanted me to stay out of it after that, but I chopped at him: "Frank, I'm going to stick with it. I'll do it whether you like it or not! You can't lock me up for that."

"You watch your step then, Russ," he said, his eyes showing concern mixed with respect. "I'll see that you get plenty of protection. We want the top man. If you find him before we do, let us know right away. No grandstanding!"

From then on I frequented the tavern where the pushers hung out, and one night the two entered. Before long a third man came in and joined them. I carried a small camera at this

THE ADJUSTMENT

time, but I needed an excuse to take a picture of the three men.

I wheeled over to a girl at the bar who seemed to be alone. "Can I buy you a beer?" I asked.

She looked at me, and I could see she felt I would be a very nontroublesome provider for an evening of free drinks.

I acted as if she had made my whole week worthwhile, and I asked her if she would mind standing across the room so that I could take a picture of her. She consented, and I placed her near the three men, then snapped the picture.

They looked surprised and scowled at me, but when they saw me return to the bar with the girl they settled back, and I imagined they figured a jerky spastic in a wheelchair was harmless.

I turned the film over to Frank, and in a few days the third man was identified. I was shocked. He was one of the math teachers at the high school. It was hard to believe he was my black king.

Frank congratulated me. "You sure did a job, Russ. Now all we have to do is put that filthy king of yours in check. A schoolteacher? It's hard to believe."

I busied myself after that, spreading the word I was a dope addict and needed a fix.

Luck? Who knows? One day one of the boys at the center said his math teacher lived on his block and that he would arrange for me to buy from him.

The arrangements were made and I set out on my mission, frightened and spastic as all get out, but I kept in mind all the boys I might be saving from a life of hell once my black king was checkmated. I was driving my special golf car. It had the most speed. I was anxious to get the buy over with. I also figured my shaking body would convince the math teacher I was truly in need of a fix. Frank had given me plenty of money to make the buy. He and his men were supposed to be nearby to witness the purchase.

I turned the corner then drove up to the teacher's house. Instead he came running out of another house with a rifle. He had learned I was helping the police.

Bullets riddled my special golf car—my Betsy. I ducked as best I could and headed for a nearby alley. Betsy, my beautiful Betsy, made the sharp turn and sped into it.

Frank and his knights jumped the black king while bishop Russell S. Schultze sat shaking and feeling himself over to make sure he was all right.

"What wonders God performs!" I thought as I sat shaking, grateful to be alive, thankful the game was over.

Frank and the others wanted to give me a special badge. I refused. "Don't give me anything—please!" I pleaded. "If Mom ever found out I did this, she'd have a stroke!"

My reward was a grand one though. Frank and my firemen friends filled Betsy's bullet holes and touched her up. My golf car was new and shiny again. Mom never found out about the adventure, and Frank insisted I get out of town for awhile.

One of my nephews packed my wheelchair into his car a few days later and drove me to Berkeley, California, to visit with Buzz and his wife, Martine.

I had a very heartwarming and interesting experience in San Francisco learning about the Orient as I traveled in style through Chinatown with two lovely Chinese girls.

12 The Big Tournament: Oriental Style

I enjoyed my visit with Buzz and his wife Martine very much, but Buzz only played checkers now, and I longed for a good tough match at the chessboard.

Buzz knew I was restless. He looked across the checkerboard one evening and said: "Russ, why don't you let me take you to Berkeley College? They have a big recreational center there, and chess is all the rage."

The next day he drove me to the college on his way to work, pulled me from the car and took me inside the recreation hall.

He slapped me on the back and said: "I'll pick you up when I'm through at work. Show these young kids over there how it's done."

I enjoyed playing with the college boys and girls, and soon I ended up giving exhibition matches, sometimes playing several students at one time, their chessboards lined up in a row, myself sitting opposite my challengers.

One day two Chinese girls approached me.

"Sir," one of them said as she bowed politely. "My cousin and I wish to play chess with you. Is this possible?"

I had more challengers than I could handle that day, but they were so delicate, so pretty, I couldn't refuse.

"Grab a couple of chessboards," I said. I ended up with six challengers instead of four.

One of the tiny Orientals opened with the P-Q4. The other opened with a P-K4, the famous Ruy Lopez opening. I lost both games to them, shocked and astonished over their ability, later finding out both their fathers were grand masters of chess, having won many international chess matches.

They showed up often at the college after that first day, still continuing to beat me at the board.

One day after I was completely exhausted from struggling to win a game with them the smaller of the two girls said: "Come with us, Russ. We'll show you Chinatown."

I wasn't prepared for such luxury as they helped me into a large red Cadillac convertible and whisked me off to San Francisco. Later I called Buzz and told him where I was.

By this time I called the tiniest girl Crackerjack, because I couldn't pronounce her given name. The other I called Wigglewalk.

The three of us got along well together, and that day they escorted me all through Chinatown in my wheelchair, showing me exotic hand-carved chess sets costing hundreds of dollars and much beautiful Chinese art.

When we returned to Berkeley, we would take our chessboards with us into restaurants while we lunched and continued with our matches. My chess improved considerably. They taught me the Koltanowski opening, and I continued to improve.

One day we were playing chess in Crackerjack's family car. She gave the chauffeur orders to drive us to her home.

I couldn't believe my eyes the first time I saw it. I was transported into another world. Beautiful low furniture spread out over the big house, and I enjoyed many fine dinners, Chinese food no restaurant could match. We sat at low tables drinking tea and talking, Crackerjack's and Wigglewalk's English far surpassing mine.

Then one day they took me to the indoor pool. Steam rose up from it.

"Get in, Russ," Crackerjack giggled. "We'll give you an Oriental bath."

They held a towel in front of me, and I slipped off my clothes ending up in my shorts.

They lifted me up and placed me in the shallow water. I

THE BIG TOURNAMENT

felt like a king that day as they cared for me.

I saw tears in Wigglewalk's eyes as she asked me how I became crippled. I told them both my story to date as they continued ministering to me.

Later they handed me a fine silk robe, and we went in to lunch.

During the fine meal, Crackerjack's father entered the room. I had briefly visited with him a few times, and he seemed to accept me into his household.

He announced they must leave for China. He had business with his brother, Wigglewalk's father.

"Father, is it possible to take Russ along?" Crackerjack asked politely.

His deep throaty command told me I would not be going to China.

The girls placed me in the family car, then paid me a great honor. My little Orientals bowed low, then backed away from the car. The chauffeur drove me back to Berkeley.

I'll always be grateful for their beautiful friendship.

That night I lay in bed thinking about San Francisco and the sights and the good times I had there, wondering what Crackerjack and Wigglewalk were doing.

"What now, Russell Schultze?" I asked, feeling sad over the separation.

I became restless after that, and a week later Buzz drove me to the bus station, and I purchased my ticket home.

When I tried to board the bus the driver said: "Sorry, but I don't take disabled people. You can't get on."

Buzz clenched his fists. "You can't do that! He bought his ticket in good faith."

"Sorry, but I can't be bothered with wheelchair cases. Now don't give me any trouble. It's my right to decide whether I want to be saddled with someone disabled. I got enough problems; now move aside!"

My money was refunded, and the next day Buzz took me to another bus line. They had a five-star general bus ticket. The ticket entitled the purchaser to sandwiches, coffee, milk, and soft drinks, and a stewardess was aboard.

We were to leave San Francisco around ten o'clock that night and head south to Los Angeles, then follow the southern route. I was to be in Moline in three days, having to change buses only two or three times. I'm sure I own the world's record on the number of times I did change buses along with the time it took me to get to Moline. I boarded twenty-one buses, the trip taking eight days.

The bus arrived in Los Angeles about five or six in the morning. I was helped from the bus and the stewardess helped me into the depot.

The ticket agent said I couldn't wait for the next bus which was due in at three o'clock that afternoon.

"The restrooms are down the basement, and there's no one to take him there. He can't stay here," she said as she glared at me.

I felt so rejected I forgot to tell her I had a urinal bottle in the sack hanging at the side of my wheelchair.

"He has to stay here!" the stewardess argued. "Where will he go?"

"Take him out!" the ticket agent shouted as the ticket window became crowded with purchasers.

I turned my chair around and headed for the door, tired and disgusted. The stewardess followed me.

"Where will you go?" she asked, concern in her voice.

"Don't worry about me," I answered. "I'll be fine. I'm used to going places by myself."

Once outside the door I steered myself down the street and entered what seemed to be an office building. The janitor was mopping the floor.

"Is there a restroom here?" I asked. I wanted to freshen up.

THE BIG TOURNAMENT 115

He stared at me for a moment, then said: "It's downstairs, but that elevator will take you down. I'll go with you and show you where it is. Then I'll come back for you in a few minutes."

When we reached the washroom, he squeezed my wheelchair together and pushed me through the narrow door.

After relieving myself and washing my face and hands, I waited for him to return. Almost an hour passed, and I knew he had forgotten about me. The only thing I could do was try to get back through the narrow door. I pushed the door open with my feet then labored trying to squeeze my wheelchair together enough to pass through the opening.

After about forty minutes of struggle I settled myself in the narrowed chair as best I could, then pushed myself through the opening, my body covered with perspiration. The long hall facing me was freedom! I didn't know which way to turn, but it didn't seem to matter. I felt I would eventually find my way out of the building.

I turned right, and as I guided my chair down the hall, the texture of the walls changed from smooth plaster to rough, and the walls were a dull grey.

I finally found an elevator and entered, pushed the button again, and the elevator went up.

The elevator door opened, and I saw a penny arcade. Next to it was a ramp, and it was too steep. My feet also became my brakes, but in spite of my pushing I almost crashed into a display.

Reaching the counter, I breathed a sigh. I had made it! A waitress asked me what I wanted. I looked up at the big board above the counter.

"I'll have a bowl of chili and a ham and cheese sandwich," I said as politely as my feelings of depression allowed.

She prepared my order and set it on the counter.

"How ya gonna eat it?" she questioned, as she looked down at me. I handed her the money.

"I'll eat it here on the stool," I answered.

"You can't do that; it isn't sanitary."

I was so tired and depressed by then that I snapped at her: "Ma'am, I will eat here! I paid for this food, and I'll eat it here! I can't climb up on that stool, so please give me my food."

"You just wait there!" she shouted, as she stormed over to the phone.

One of the customers took pity on me and picked my order up as I placed the napkin on the stool. He set it on the napkin.

The waitress returned. "I said you couldn't eat on that stool!"

"It's working pretty good," I answered.

She leaned over the counter to pick up my bowl of chili.

"Look, lady," I said, "just leave me alone! I'll give you back your bowl."

A policeman entered, and the waitress shouted, "That's him! I told him he couldn't eat on that stool. It's against the law!"

"What law?" the policeman asked, as he smiled at me.

"Never mind, Officer," I said. "I'm not too hungry anyway."

I took the remains of my sandwich and spun the wheelchair around and left.

There was a gift shop next to the coffee shop, and I entered it as I nibbled at my sandwich, choking back my loneliness. I slowly moved about trying to dispel my feelings, examining a miniature chess set and several other interesting items.

The lady clerk came up to me. "Sir, I'll have to take a look in that bag at the side of your wheelchair."

"She thinks I'm a thief," I thought. I was so tired and discouraged by then I shouted: "You most certainly will not! You'll have to get a search warrant!"

I guided my chair toward the door. "I'll be outside on the corner. You call the police if you like; I'll be waiting!"

I hated Los Angeles by then and thought: "The City of Angels." I laughed. "The big City of Angels!"

I steered my wheelchair vigorously to the corner. "Where's

the bus station?" I thought as my muscles shook and my head bobbed. The heavy traffic also made my head spin.

I discovered the bus station was across the street. I had passed under the street from one building to another.

The traffic frightened me, and I asked several people to help me get back across the street. They all passed me by.

I spotted a policeman and approached him. "Would you please help me across the street? I have a bus to catch."

He looked down at me. "I'm too busy; just got a call." He stepped into his squad car and drove away.

I remembered Frank back in Moline, choked back my tears, and spoke to the busy street. "Frank wouldn't ever do such a thing to someone."

I don't think I ever felt so alone as the traffic rushed by me, people walking around my wheelchair as I sat by the curb. I had drawn a stalemate. I couldn't go across the street by myself with four lanes of traffic rushing by.

"O God!" I cried. "Doesn't anybody want to help me?"

I saw a cab approaching and waved him down. He stopped.

I stammered: "I have . . . to . . . catch a bus. I'll . . . pay you if you help me across the street."

He got out of the cab and helped me across.

"What's the charge?" I asked.

"A buck will do," he answered as he stood jingling the coins in his pocket.

I would have gladly paid him five at the time. I was safe at last, and the bus station was only a few doors down. I backed my chair up against a building to escape the chilling air, took off my cap, and closed my eyes. Soon I dozed off.

Suddenly I felt something land in my cap, opened my eyes, and someone had tossed a quarter into it.

"Now I'm a beggar!" I cried. "Just a beggar!"

My afternoon in Los Angeles was complete after a poorly dressed man with healthy red cheeks came up to me on crutches.

"Look, buddy," he lashed out. "Get out of here! This has been my corner for years. If you don't get out, I'll wrap that wheelchair around your neck; now scram!"

"Look mister," I said as my head bobbed and my body shook, "I'm only trying to take a nap. I have a bus to catch."

"Then catch it!" he shouted as he kicked my wheelchair with his bandaged foot.

I swung the chair around and went inside the bus station. It was crowded, and the ticket agent glared at me. I left.

Down the street I spotted a small restaurant and entered. A man left the cash register and came up to me. "Come in," he said politely. He showed me to a table. "Want a menu?"

"I-have-a-bus-to-catch-soon, and-I-would-like-some-milk," I said, hearing my choppy voice.

He brought the milk to me, but I was so nervous that I spilled it all over the table and the floor.

His smile was beautiful. "There's more where that came from. How about a straw?"

"That-will-be-fine," I stammered as he mopped up my mess.

He returned with the milk and the straw and sat down opposite me. I told him my tale of woe.

"Ya got to learn to roll with the punches, buddy," he lectured. "Ya got to know that everybody has problems and forgive 'em. This helps when things get rough."

Later he took me to the washroom and helped me to the urinal, holding me while I relieved myself.

I wasn't charged for the milk, and I accepted his hospitality and thanked him, knowing I would be less than gracious if I insisted on paying.

My bus finally arrived, and I was placed on board trouble free. An ex-soldier and an English girl were very kind to me, helping me at bus changes until we reached St. Louis.

From St. Louis to Moline I experienced the bulk of my bus

changes as the smaller buses either developed flat tires or broke down.

The bus finally pulled into the Moline depot. My sister Snooky stood beside it. She was a beautiful sight. I was home!

After I was helped from the bus and placed in my wheelchair, Snooky kissed me. I thought how wonderful it is to be loved! Then I remembered the few in Los Angeles who had cared.

It was then that I decided my life would be spent helping others. For the rest of my life, I decided, I would continue helping Frank with his kids of the streets. I didn't know I would be swept into deep sorrow the following day.

13 Circuit Breaker: Loss—New Light— Then Love

The following morning was warm, the leaves coated with splashes of color as Mother Nature painted her autumn scene. I was anxious to see Frank, Pete, and my other firemen friends.

I reached the fire station and entered through the open doors. Pete saw me and came over.

"How was the trip, Russ?"

"All right, I guess," I answered. "Has Frank been here yet?"

Pete looked at the floor and shoved his hands into his pockets. "I'm sorry, Russ, but Frank is dead. He died while on duty—heart attack."

I became immersed in sorrow, staring at the bloodred fire truck as the morning sun made shiny ripples on the hood. All I could think about was my sorrow. Pete went to get me a cup of coffee.

I looked out onto the street. Two boys were approaching the station, boys I remembered I had helped at one time, and I thought, "I'll always help your boys, Frank."

As the boys passed the station, their shadows fell across the hood of the fire engine. They saw me sitting beside it.

"Hey, Russ! When did you get back into town?" one of them said.

They came into the station, and the smiles on their faces were uplifting, easing some of my sorrow. They looked like angels to me that day, and I smiled back. "Want to play some chess?" I asked, my tears I'm sure making my eyes as shiny as the old truck beside me.

"Sure do," they answered with interest. At that moment the boys were no longer Frank's kids of the streets; they were mine.

The circuit was broken, and I knew I must bury my sorrow and help the boys and girls Frank had cared so much about.

This became difficult, however. My father retired soon after that and built a house in Coal Valley, a small town near Moline. I had far to travel but managed to get to the civic center in Rock Island because I received a small pension as a dependent now and this paid for my gas.

After only a few years in Coal Valley my father died of a heart attack.

After the funeral services at the cemetery, I looked up and viewed the blue sky, white clouds hanging from it like a shroud. My thoughts drifted with those clouds back to the hospital in Chicago. I recalled the early morning experience I had with my grandfather as we watched the earth separate, one half of it drifting into the large white cloud. That memory comforted me that day, for I took heart that Dad was with Grandfather Sears, Mary Ellen, and Frank.

Later Mom was at a loss for what to do with her life, and after many frustrating weeks she decided to sell the house. We moved back to Moline next door to my sister Snooky who was married by then.

It wasn't long after the move that it was discovered I had an ulcer. It grew worse, and I ended up in the hospital. The prognosis was not good, and I longed to see my family in California. Snooky flew there with me.

Once there, I sat in the warm sun visiting with Buzz, Pete, Toots, and their families—Snooky seeing to my diet and medication, and the love and attention helped restore my health I'm sure. I grew stronger each day and thanked God for my recovery.

One afternoon I was lying in the hammock resting, and I again thought about my experience at the hospital in Chicago when my grandfather told me I must learn more about my Master.

When I returned to Moline with Snooky, I visited many

CIRCUIT BREAKER

churches and continued to help my kids of the streets.

Soon after my return I also had a visitor, a man whom I had helped once. He had moved away and returned to the Quad Cities.

He opened up a case of household products and handed me some charts. "Why don't you sign up with me? We'll both be rich, Russ."

I was a doubting Thomas. The products sounded too good to be true. He pointed to one of the special items.

"I see you have a bad rash, Russ. I'll give you baths in this famous detergent cure-all."

I laughed, knowing there hadn't been anything that helped the skin rash I had developed along with the ulcer.

He ministered to me often after that. As the weeks passed there was much improvement. He took me to one of the sales meetings, and I was sold on the company and its products. He became my sponsor, and we were in business. I was finally able to support myself. It was a wonderful feeling.

However, my friend was never one to stay with anything for long. He left town, and I was turned over to another sponsor. His name was Jim Moser.

Jim Moser and his wife Andrea became very dear friends of mine. One evening they introduced me to the minister of their church. I attended church with them after that, and the minister, Donald G. Hunt, was the best teacher of the Bible I had ever known. His sermons brought to me what I had been searching for all my life, it seemed. I found a stronger faith through Brother Hunt. He is a brilliant man and has written and published several textbooks on Bible study. He has also edited *The Voice of Evangelism* since 1946, and has taught in Midwestern School of Evangelism at Ottumwa, Iowa. He has been an evangelist since 1942.

I became so taken with Brother Hunt I joined his church. During my baptismal immersion, as I lay beneath the water, I looked up into Brother Hunt's face. The serenity I saw there was transformed to the very heart of me. I remembered the time at the hospital when I was thirteen as I lay drowning beneath the tub of water, praying for faith—the faith of a mustard seed. As I looked into Brother Hunt's face, I knew I had that faith.

I was taken from the water and felt clean—pure. Even though I had prayed for forgiveness of my sins many times, I had never truly felt the Lord had forgiven me. That night I knew he had! I was truly happy.

I continued selling my household products along with giving chess lessons and visiting Jim Moser and his wife Andrea. They were a happy couple, and I wished I had a life like theirs.

One day I said to Andrea: "I'm lonesome. I wish I had a wife. I can support one now. You and Jim are so happy together. It must be wonderful."

She smiled and said: "Ask the Lord. He always grants us what is right in his eyes."

I went home and prayed fervently for a life's companion. A few weeks later I received a phone call. The voice was soft and pleasing

"Hello, is this Mr. Schultze—Russell Schultze?"

"Yes," I answered.

"My name is Kathy Bestian. Your name was given to me through the Cerebral Palsy Foundation. There is to be a social club for all handicapped people. We're just starting, and we're calling the new club the 'Handi-capables.' Would you like to join?"

During the conversation I asked how old she was.

"How old are you, Mr. Schultze?" she questioned.

I swallowed hard. "I'm . . . I'm . . . forty-nine."

She hesitated a moment. Then I heard her chuckle. "I'm thirty-seven and holding."

I liked her sense of humor. I wanted to see her.

"When's the meeting?" I asked expectantly. "You had better give me your phone number so I can let you know."

CIRCUIT BREAKER

"The meeting is at the Butterworth Center in Moline the week of June 6, at 7:00 P.M.," she said. Then she gave me her number.

"I'll probably be there if the weather permits. I drive an open golf car," I announced, hoping the weather would be nice.

"Oh!" she exclaimed, her voice telling me she was impressed. "You're the one who rides all over town in that car. I saw you once or twice some time ago, and I have been wanting to meet you ever since. I hope you can make it to the meeting."

I felt my blood pressure rise. She wanted to meet me! I had to see her! Then I heard the click and sighed. The circuit was broken, but I knew I would be going to the meeting come rain or shine.

14 Heavens to Betsy: New Life—New Responsibilities

June 6, the day of the "Handi-capable" meeting, arrived. It was a beautiful day. As I looked out my bedroom window, Mom's early roses nodded in the breeze.

After two hours of meticulous preparation, the old swain sat in front of the mirror inspecting himself like a field marshal inspecting troops on parade. Was I kidding myself? Would I make a fool of myself? Then I felt shame. Had I lost faith again? Had I forgotten the many Bible passages Brother Hunt so expertly explained in his fine books and sermons? Then I saluted the sandy-haired, blue-eyed man in the mirror with renewed faith, swirled my wheelchair around, and pushed myself from the room.

Mom came into the hall. "I'm eating out tonight, Mom. I won't be home for dinner. I have lots of deliveries to make. Then I'm going to a meeting at the Butterworth Center."

"What's going on there?" she asked. "My, you do look nice, Russ."

"The meeting is about a new club for handicapped people. I'm going to join."

She smiled and patted me on the head as though I were still her little boy. "That sounds like something very worthwhile. Have a nice time; but don't stay out too late."

I was anxious to meet Kathy Bestian, and my movements were a little too swift as I approached the front door. I pushed my foot right through the screen.

As I came to my golf car, I patted my Betsy's shiny hood, then struggled onto one of her soft seats, took the ropes I had rigged up, and tied them to the wheelchair. I maneuvered the ropes, and soon the chair was securely strapped to Betsy's side. Then we were off down the alley toward the street.

"Please, Lord," I prayed, "don't let Betsy break down today. I want to go to that meeting clean and not covered with grease." Then I frowned, thinking about the times she had broken down. When she wasn't in tip-top shape, I didn't feel good either. But she performed as I had never known her to do, purring all through my many deliveries.

I arrived at the civic center an hour early and sat wondering how the evening would turn out. I didn't know what Kathy Bestian looked like. How would I find her? Then I remembered she had seen me a couple of times. Would she recognize me?

A man parked in back of Betsy and stepped from his car. He helped me with my wheelchair, and soon I was inside the center. Others began to arrive. I watched them enter the fine old house which the prominent Mrs. Butterworth had donated as a civic center.

Then a beautiful blond made a grand entrance, a handsome man pushing her through the door.

She came nearer, then raised her delicate soft hand in a queenly gesture for her escort to stop. My heart thumped as she smiled at me. Her eyes were blue, and she looked like a Dresden doll, her white ruffled blouse framing her lovely face. Then her soft-looking lips parted.

"Are you Russell Schultze? I'm Kathy Bestian."

"Yes . . . I . . . am," I answered, feeling a tightening in my throat.

She looked only eighteen or twenty instead of thirty-seven. She was beautiful!

"This is my friend, Vic," she announced.

I had hoped the man escorting her was her brother or cousin. He presented a threat to me, but his warm welcome told me he could never become an enemy or anything closely resembling one.

Then he pushed her to the center of the room now crowded with wheelchairs supporting the many who seemed anxious for companionship.

I inched my way through the crowd until I reached her side. The meeting began, and the first order of the evening was a get-acquainted session. Names of famous people or places were pinned to our backs, and we were to ask each other questions in order to discover the name or place we were supposed to be.

After questioning Kathy about my name tag I discovered I was Bobby Fischer, the famous chess player. She was supposed to be Elizabeth Taylor, but I thought her far more beautiful than the lovely Liz. I wanted so desperately to see her again, and I quickly devised a plan that would include her in a social gathering. I invited the whole group to a potluck picnic.

Peggy, one of the leaders, made the announcement toward the end of the evening, and I made sure Kathy would attend. However, as I drove home that night, I was disturbed. I had discovered that the girl of my prayers lived eighteen miles from Moline. This meant if I ever did get the chance to call on her it would take me at least an hour and a half to get there. Then I remembered my Betsy could travel almost fifty miles on a gallon of gas. I would have enough money left over to take Kathy to many fine places if she would only consent to go with me.

The next day I decided to call her. I felt I had to find out what interested her most. This would be a beginning at least. To my amazement I found she was an Olympic star of sorts. She had at one time joined "The Rough Riders," a wheelchair basketball team in the area, and had won third place ribbons in javelin and discus throwing. This was my delicate Kathy?

My Dresden doll? I couldn't even throw myself out of a wheelchair successfully. She didn't play chess. The only common ground I discovered was her great interest in my Betsy. I thanked heaven I had my little car.

The next day I set out for the town of Taylor Ridge. It took me over two hours to get there, asking directions, and then making wrong turns due to my anxiety.

When I reached her parent's farm, I drove into the yard, honked, and her dad pushed her out of the door and down a very short ramp. I thought at the time if she had a longer ramp she could have managed on her own. I found out later she was waited on too much—even by the housekeeper after her mother died, and I knew this was not good for her. She would be happier if she did more things for herself.

Her hair that day was golden in the sunlight, and her eyes matched the sky.

"This is Russell Schultze, Dad," she said.

He looked at me, and I could see he was concerned. I guess I didn't look like a man who could take proper care of her, and he eyed my Betsy with scorn as her wide tires pressed into his beautifully kept lawn.

"Would you like to go for a drive, Kathy?" I asked.

Her father's eyes told me he wasn't too happy about it. Then he scratched his chin and searched my car over.

"If you came all the way out here from Moline without being killed, I guess it's all right if she goes for a little ride." He picked her up and placed her in the car beside me.

"Are you all right?" I asked as the car bounced over the lawn, Betsy's tires making marks on the freshly cut grass. I had never taken a paraplegic in my car before, and I was worried.

"Yes, this is fine," she answered excitedly.

I could see she wanted to get her hand on the steering bar. I would have an excuse to hold it!

"Would you like to drive?" I asked.

"Oh!" she exclaimed. "Do you think I could?"

"Sure," I answered, "just put your hand on the steering bar here." She did, and mine closed over hers. I slowly squeezed the soft flesh, feeling the blood race faster through my veins. Then I showed her how to steer after setting the gearshift in low, not trusting the enthusiasm I saw in her eyes.

She did very well until she spotted her sister-in-law who lived on the next farm. She waved, and I had forgotten to tell her how to stop on an incline. She took her other hand off the steering bar, and the car headed for a ditch.

I grabbed the hand brake and struggled to put the car in reverse.

"Be patient with me," I said. "It takes me longer to calm down than most people."

After I removed Betsy from the peril Kathy had placed her in, I looked at the blond beauty beside me and smiled a forgiving smile.

"I didn't do too badly, did I?" she asked with an apologetic tone in her voice.

"No, you did fine," I lied. "You did just fine!"

Our first picnic was stormy. Drops of rain fell throughout the afternoon, and I was upset because Vic had accompanied Kathy there. He seemed to be quite a "Handi-capable" helper, and I was worried. I could see Kathy thought a lot of him.

I took several of the picnickers for a ride around the park, and after awhile I asked Kathy if she wanted to ride.

"Of course," she answered. "I thought you would never ask. Vic, put me in the car."

He did her bidding, and after a few turns around the park I drove out the gate.

"I want you to meet my mother," I said with a significant raise of my eyebrows.

"We had better not be too long," she answered. "Vic might not like it."

I drove her around my neighborhood and introduced her as my girlfriend. She blushed. I knew I was rushing things, but I didn't care.

Mom was not pleased, but the rest of the family was delighted to meet Kathy. She sat proud as a princess, but her right leg kept slipping over the edge of the car from time to time. This worried me. I didn't want her to get hurt, and I mentioned it to Snooky. She went into her house and brought out an old nylon stocking and tied Kathy's legs to my right one.

"Now you've tied the knot," Snooky joked. I blushed along with Kathy.

After driving around a short while longer, we returned to the picnic. Kathy's friend Vic was waiting for her. He wasn't angry with me, and I wished the afternoon could go on forever even though the light rain had turned into a torrent.

As our courtship progressed, Kathy and I became interested in the bowling the other "Handi-capables" were involved in, and to my amazement I found I did quite well. We bowled from a special ramp at one of the bowling alleys, and this new interest helped our friendship grow. Kathy became exceptionally good at bowling, almost reaching the lofty heights of a two hundred game. I was very proud of her.

That winter our phone conversations became a big part of our courtship because of the weather and the distance between us. We learned many things about each other.

I told her all about myself and about Mary Ellen. I cried that night as I recalled my first love.

Kathy told me about her condition. When she was fourteen she had a strep throat which led to a spinal disease that left her paralyzed from the waist down. She began to cry when she told me about a boy she had loved. He was burned in a fire, and the shock had made her think about ending her life with sleeping pills.

I soothed, "Look, honey, I'm awfully glad you didn't die.

We wouldn't be here talking like this if you had. Please don't cry. As soon as the roads clear, I'll come out and we'll be together again."

Spring came, and we were happy as we drove over country roads or went to drive-in movies or bowled.

I knew I loved her by then, but I wasn't sure she truly loved me.

I busied myself with plans to build a longer ramp at her farm so she could get outside by herself. Her father seemed to resent it so I stopped. He seemed to resent everything I did to help her be more independent. I guess he didn't want to lose her, or perhaps he felt I couldn't take proper care of her. We continued to see each other in spite of everything.

Then one night I said to Mom: "I'm about to get myself engaged."

Her face turned white, and she said: "How did this woman manage to do this to you?"

"Mom," I answered, "it's not her idea. It's mine! I love her, and I want to get married."

She placed her hands on her hips defiantly and walked out of the room. As I was eating my supper by the television, I heard her sniffles and knew she was very upset. I was, too. Mom and Kathy's dad were keeping us apart. They didn't trust us to marriage. I prayed about the situation and felt a determination sweep over me. We would be married!

After that night I fretted over where we would live if we did marry. Could I find an apartment I could afford?

Then one day my wonderful sister Snooky came into my room. She lived next door at the time.

"Russ," she said, with a finality in her voice, "Mom is in her eighties, and you must live your own life. My family took a vote last night, and it was unanimous that you convert our double garage and breezeway into living quarters. We'll all help. You go ahead with your marriage."

I was so happy. I would still be near Mom. I wouldn't feel I had deserted her. I could still be on hand to help her and give her the companionship she was used to.

After Snooky left I called Kathy and asked her point blank to marry me.

"Yes, I guess so," was her answer.

I could tell by her voice she had mixed emotions. I told her about Snooky's offer. "We'll have a nice place of our own."

She hesitated for awhile. "Let me think about it, Russ. Call me tomorrow."

I called her the next day and said, "Is this my future wife?" I felt as cold and clammy as a salmon that had flopped onto a bank and couldn't get back to safe water. Even my pet ulcer turned flip-flops as I waited for her answer.

"You're a sneaky character rushing me into a yes, but it's yes!"

The day of our wedding Kathy looked like an angel as she came down the aisle, her brother-in-law, Tom, pushing her wheelchair, her father walking along beside her.

Kathy's friend Vic stood in attendance along with my best man, Kenny, one of my nephews.

I felt like all heaven was looking down upon us that day as we listened to our vows. I glanced over at my bride, and her face told me everything was right and good.

After the usual reception, greeting our friends, and enjoying the beautiful traditional cake, Kathy and I, along with Buzz and my nephew Kenny, drove home.

When we reached the alley and drove into the yard, I looked at the haven that had been created by me and our friends. I was proud. We had a home of our own!

Buzz carried each of us into the double garage dwelling, and after our many well-wishing friends and relatives left, the woman I married looked at me, a soft blush on her beautiful face.

Then she quietly wheeled herself around the corner of the

breezeway which had been turned into a bathroom of sorts.

It seemed it took me an hour before I managed to slip into my pajamas.

Then Kathy entered the main part of our house wrapped in a beautiful pink negligee, her golden hair falling onto her shoulders. She seemed calm and smiled at me. Then she removed the foot rests from her wheelchair in order to get closer to the bed.

"Careful now," I cautioned. I felt so inadequate. After much struggling she flopped onto the bed, pale, and exhausted.

I tipped my own wheelchair backward, and after pushing with all my might I also ended up safely on the bed, grateful I hadn't ended up on the floor, I was so nervous.

"How about a game of chess?" I asked as we lay breathless.

She laughed and pushed herself nearer to me. "No, Mr. Schultze. You'll have to think of something else. I didn't marry you for your ability at the chessboard."

I took her in my arms, and after much trial and error we discovered we were far more than just two people who needed companionship. We discovered many secrets that night along with the sensitive spot behind Kathy's ear and the way she responded. Love came quite naturally to us that night, and we reveled in the glory of it.

It wasn't too long before my lady conquered her household tasks from her wheelchair. Her duties took her ten times as long to perform as they would a normal housewife, and cooking was difficult for her, because soon after our marriage we discovered she had a diabetic condition, and of course, my ulcer misbehaved at times. Often she groaned over the many dishes she had to prepare, but she always looked at me apologetically and smiled.

We were happy; very happy. But as the old saying goes: "In every life a little rain must fall," some did fall on our newly formed household.

Kathy and I went to a drive-in movie one night. I wasn't feeling very well, and she had a headache. We left, and when we entered the house I felt the fullness in my throat.

"Get me a pan—quick!" I gurgled.

She hurried to the sink and returned with a pan. I grabbed it just as the blood gushed from my mouth. I ended up in the hospital with my bleeding ulcer, and naturally Kathy was teased unmercifully about her cooking.

We spent our first month's anniversary with Kathy visiting me at the hospital. Then I was released and ready to take on responsibility again.

We enjoyed the neighborhood children very much. They helped Kathy with some of her chores, and I taught some of them chess. I showed the older boys in the neighborhood my engines, and it wasn't long before they were interested in mechanics. They helped me work on my two cars.

Our second month of marriage was also traumatic, though. The only good thing about that month was the fact that the electric hoist for over the bed arrived. Kathy and I wouldn't have to struggle to get into bed anymore.

One morning I raised myself up and managed to lay in the strap attached to the hoist. I was on my stomach and began to swing back and forth.

"Come on, Peter Pan," Kathy laughed, as she gave me an extra push. "Let's get moving; I'm hungry."

After an hour and a half of bathing beside the sink at one side of the bed and dressing ourselves, we were ready for the day.

"Ladies first," I said as I helped place the strap beneath Kathy. She was lifted up and away from me, the hoist carrying her to the foot of the bed and gently placing her in her wheelchair.

She set the machine in motion again, and soon we were seated at the table over poached eggs and toast.

"Want to go for a ride?" I said. "It's a beautiful fall day." I turned and looked out of the picture window at the front of the garage. The leaves were red and gold, the grass still green from summer. It was beautiful. Our morning prayer included a thank-you for the fine weather.

"Let's take Suzy along. She likes hamburgers," Kathy answered. "We'll drive all afternoon and then stop at a drive-in for supper."

Suzy was our little neighbor girl. We loved her very much and thought of her as our own.

"Sure, honey," I agreed, as I thought about the beautiful afternoon ahead of us.

We drove through town, enjoying the well-kept lawns, still free from dead leaves that soon would lay limp beneath the snow.

It was getting late, and we were hungry. We headed for the nearest drive-in.

As I made a left turn I didn't see the on-coming car. The car struck my Betsy just ahead of the front seat on Kathy's side. I lost my shoe. Our legs were hanging over the sides of the car. Little Suzy was in the backseat.

I turned around as best I could. "You all right, honey?" I thanked God she was as she answered a startled yes.

Kathy sat stunned. "You didn't see him," she said, and her voice sounded as if it were coming from inside a deep well.

The man who had hit us got out of his car and approached us. He looked us over, and his eyes rested upon my dangling leg. "Your leg looks crooked. I think it's broken," he announced.

"Put my shoe back on," I said. I felt the pain as he pushed the shoe onto my foot. "I broke my leg all right," I winced.

Kathy started to cry. People were crowded around us, and soon I heard the ambulance.

At the hospital I was treated for the broken leg and remained. Kathy was checked over and X-rayed.

She came into my room before she left the hospital. She

was in tears, and I didn't want that. I was lying in bed, my leg in a cast. "Gee whiz," I said, as cheerfully as I could. "Now I can't play Peter Pan for awhile."

She leaned toward me, but the bed kept her from the kiss she tried to deliver.

"It will all be over soon, honey," I said as I praised the Lord things weren't worse. She smiled through her tears, wheeled herself to the door, and left, too sad to look back, I'm sure.

After she was home, her right leg began to swell. She was brought back to the hospital and X-rayed again. The leg was broken. She also ended up in the hospital, and we were placed in separate rooms, but the nurses were very kind and saw that we ate together. We also visited each other often.

One day Kathy banged her tiny fist down on my bed. "Look at us! We look like a pair of bookends."

Our sense of humor returned, and we laughed. We spent our days together planning what we would do when we left the hospital.

We returned home, both in our casts, friends and relatives helping with some of the chores. Eleven-year-old Suzy was also on hand to help out.

After that things went along well until one day, as I was putting up my orders, I smelled smoke. It was close by, and it smelled like burning hair. I couldn't understand it until I heard a sound like popcorn popping in a popper. I looked down, and I saw the puffs of smoke. "My electric wheelchair's on fire! A short in the wiring!" I yelled.

I sat like a condemned man waiting for the final jolt as the old chair popped and sputtered.

Little Suzy squealed and ran from the house. She returned with my niece Karen, and Karen, Suzy, and Kathy dragged me from the burning wheelchair and placed me into an older one. They frantically pushed the popping, cracking electric chair out the door into the yard.

When the fire truck arrived, I hailed my firemen friends, nervously waving my arms. The yard was beginning to fill with concerned neighbors, and Kathy's sister drove up.

"Are things getting too dull for you folks?" she teased. She looked at the firemen. "You must be Russ's friends he's always talking about."

"Not us," one of them said. "He's trouble!" Then he waved to me. "Hey, Russ, if you have any more problems, call the police!"

"Can't!" I hollered back. "They were just here this morning yelling at me about getting some insurance and a license."

This seemed to be the end of our troubles, and that winter the organization Fish, Inc. was always prompt when Kathy or I needed a ride to the doctor or dentist. It is truly a blessed organization.

The following August of '75 I was privileged to attend the national chess tournament at Lincoln, Nebraska. Kathy had a chance to visit her sister Shirley in Kentucky.

Needless to say, I didn't win in the nationals. And memories of Lincoln returned. I missed Kathy and called her up. She was lonesome, too. We knew we had to return home. By then we were so wrapped up in each other nothing else seemed to matter.

Then one night she made me happier than I had ever been. I had prayed for the day she might decide to join my church. Our good friend Deeny, also handicapped, was being immersed that evening.

Kathy leaned over and said: "I'm going to be baptized too, Russ."

I reached over, my shaking hand squeezing hers. "Kathy, oh, Kathy," was all I could say.

Later that evening as she was placed in the water I cried tears of joy.

Our life after that seemed to settle into a mood of complete understanding and happiness, and it was all anyone could ask for.

Up to this point Mom had seemed to keep her distance. But soon after Kathy's baptism Mom changed.

It was a Sunday night. Kathy and I had been to church services. We entered our double garage castle, and Kathy had prepared ahead of time a fine chicken dinner. We invited Mom.

Mom sat down gingerly, and her expert eyes took in the well-laid table. I could see she was favorably impressed. I watched while she and Kathy chatted comfortably, and I said a silent prayer of thanksgiving. After Mom left I helped Kathy straighten up.

Bedtime came, and Kathy took the hooks on the lift and attached them to the strap beneath her. The special hoist lifted her up and away toward the bed. The motor stopped while she was in midair.

"Something's wrong," she groaned.

I wheeled myself over to the bed. "Must be trouble in the switch," I said confidently. "I'll fix it, honey."

I hurried to my tool bench and grabbed up a wrench along with some other tools.

"Hurry up," she moaned. "My upper back is getting tired."

"Don't panic, honey. I'll get you down; I promise!"

Tipping my wheelchair backward, I pushed with my elbows until I landed on the bed.

"Heaven's to Betsy, Russ," she said, with tears in her eyes. "Why does everything have to happen to us?"

"We're not the only ones, Kathy," I said sharply. "Remember that!"

Then I started to shake and bit my lip. Becoming more spastic wouldn't bring me closer to her, and I forced my mind to command my body. Soon I became more calm and went to work on the hoist. After many frustrating yanks and turns, along with tightening some screws, I was ready to try the switch. I turned it back on, and there was silence. I had failed!

"What now, Russell Schultze?" she scolded, a disgusted look on her pretty Dresden face.

I looked up at her and smiled.

"What ever comes, Kathy, our faith in God and our love for each other will make it right."

I took the strap which held her from me and then with the other hand I pushed at her bottom, releasing some of the weight on the strap, unhooked it, then rolled over as she came bouncing down onto the mattress.

She screamed; then we laughed as we lay beside each other, our laughter ringing throughout our single room dwelling.

I took her in my arms and kissed her, gently rubbing the sensitive spot behind her ear.

She giggled and snuggled closer to me, her lips brushing my face.

"Russell Schultze," she teased, "you should write a book; you really should!"

My arms tightened about her, and I sighed: "Maybe someday somebody will, Kathy love, maybe they will."